Our NHS is CRASHING

An Examination of the Rationale for HealthCRASH & its Mitigation

By Andrew J Vincent

What Others Are Saying (Already)

"Compelling and challenging - this powerful little book will help clarify your thinking on where our NHS is heading. Recommended!"

Dr Mark Newbold (Doctor and Senior Manager)

"Change always starts with clarifying and accepting the truth of a situation. If you are genuinely concerned that the NHS is in crisis, this is the place to start."

Dr Steve Allder (Consultant Neurologist)

"A must read for anyone serious about the future of the NHS and General Practice, this book concisely and logically examines the evidence and sets out the tools individuals and organisations need to survive and thrive into the future."

Paul Conroy (Practice Manager)

To Sara

I would like to dedicate this book, despite its rather austere contents, to my wife, Sara.

Quite apart from her supreme tolerance of losing me to a keyboard as frequently as she does, she inspires me in so many ways, whilst challenging me in all of the best ways.

Regardless of her own pressures, she approaches every day with enthusiasm and gusto, always with time for others.

She is an example of what makes our NHS so great and why I feel so passionately about contributing to making it work. She is not the only example, of course, but she is my very special one.

TABLE OF CONTENTS

AND SO WE BEGIN **8**

A VITAL BEHAVIOURAL INTRODUCTION **10**

THE DANGER OF DENIAL 10

THE LIMBIC PROCESSING TRAP 12

ANALYSING OUR CIRCUMSTANCES **15**

SIMPLE CONCEPTUAL FRAMEWORK 16

A FINAL WORD OF CAUTION & REASSURANCE 17

HOW WE'LL EXAMINE HEALTHCRASH LIKELIHOOD............................19

Q1. ARE THE CHALLENGES BIG ENOUGH....................................**20**

POPULATION...20

Sources of Population Data *23*

ECONOMICS..23

Sources of Economic Information *28*

CARE COMPLEXITY 30

ADVANCES..32

IN SUMMARY OF OUR 4 HORSEMEN 34

Q2. EVIDENCE OF A SYSTEM IN DECLINE....................................**36**

FINANCIAL DECLINE 36

OPERATIONAL DECLINE 40

Accident & Emergency...*40*

Elective Treatment...*41*

Cancer Referrals...*44*

In Summary of Operational Decline..*46*

QUALITY DECLINE 48

DECLINE IN MORALE..55

IN SUMMARY OF QUESTION 2 63

Q3. A QUESTION OF CAPABILITY **65**

WIDER LOSS OF CAPABILITY 66

INSUFFICIENT ENABLEMENT 68

Starting with WILL *70*

Examining SKILL...*71*

What about CAPACITY? 73

And Finally, AUTHORITY 75

IMPOSSIBLE CONDITIONS 77

IN SUMMARY OF OUR CAPABILITY 83

Q4. WHO ARE THE RESCUERS? 85

THE GOVERNMENT AS RESCUER 85

ANOTHER GOVERNMENT AS RESCUER 88

THE POPULATION AS RESCUER 89

WHAT ABOUT COMMERCIAL RESCUERS? 90

IS HEALTHCRASH A LIKELIHOOD? 93

COULD WE STILL PREVENT HEALTHCRASH? 95

Introducing Leadership Potency 96

Preventing HealthCRASH 102

A MOMENT OF REFLECTION 108

An Important Personal Moment 110

GUIDANCE ON FACING HEALTHCRASH 112

GIVE FISH OR TEACH FISHING? 113

THREE TYPES OF MITIGATION 116

WHAT ACTUALLY IS HEALTHCRASH? 118

The Dark Side of HealthCRASH 121

UPGRADING OUR LEVEL OF UNDERSTANDING 124

E1 - Protecting What You Shouldn't 125

E2 - Ignoring the New Specification 126

E3 - Seeing Things Simplistically 127

E4 - Behaving with Authority 128

E5 - Failing to Seize Opportunity 130

A Critical Need 132

The Individual Component 135

ORGANISATIONAL RESPONSES & GUIDANCE 137

DISASTER AVERSION 139

Rapid Adaptability 139

The Service-led Organisation 141

Vital Clinical Mitigation 144

Financial Mitigation..*146*

DISASTER PREPARATION *149*

Mental Preparation *149*

Leadership Readiness...*151*

Organisational Readiness Plan *152*

DISASTER RECOVERY - A FUTURE VIEW...*157*

The People Component of Recovery *158*

Reiterating Service-led & Adaptability...*160*

Readiness for a New System...*160*

Accountable Care Organisations *162*

Owned by the Innovators..*167*

In Summary of Recovery *169*

INDIVIDUAL RESPONSES & GUIDANCE **172**

REFLECTING ON PERSONAL CONSEQUENCES *173*

Health & Well-being Consequences..*173*

Professional Consequences...*175*

DISASTER AVERSION *177*

Challenge Poor Choices & Strategies *177*

Promote Good Thinking & Practice...*179*

Contribute Positively to Good Organisations..................................*182*

Health & Wellbeing Disaster Aversion...*185*

Employment & Career Disaster Aversion..*190*

DISASTER PREPARATION *194*

The Plan B Approach..*195*

Financial Preparation..*196*

Emotional Preparation...*199*

DISASTER RECOVERY...*201*

Preserving Recovery Faculties..*202*

Recovery Networks *205*

IN OVERALL SUMMARY **208**

WHAT NEXT GUIDANCE...**211**

ABOUT THE AUTHOR...**213**

And So We Begin

The title represents a bold claim that many would regard as alarmist or sensationalist. And yet, I am prone to neither tendency. What's more, after carefully observing and examining our healthcare system, its policies, provider responses and behaviour, regulators and their collective results for more than a decade, a decade that has been filled with disaster predictions that haven't previously prompted this conclusion from me when I look in depth, here I am making exactly that prediction now and it's a shorter term prediction, not a long term one.

Even now you will be developing a reaction and you've pretty much only had the title so far. It will probably come in an 'agree' or 'disagree' form in your mind. You may even develop mental antibodies to the title.

I am going to ask you one question, regardless of whether your current, immediate reaction is to discount this conclusion or agree with it. That question is this; to what degree is your reaction or conclusion based on a detached, objective analysis of the data, behaviours and myriad of factors at play, engaged in without emotional bias, reflected on, tested and supported by evidence?

For most individuals it is simple that - a reaction, without substance, evidence or proper reflection. And yet, this is your life and career that could be impacted, as well as the lives of co-workers, patients and public at large. Nobody should ask that you conclude something specific but, given the implications, don't you owe it to yourself and all to ensure you, regardless of anybody else's failure to do the same, take the trouble to think more deeply about it?

Depending on that reflection, I am going to ask you what you think you should 'do' in response. I would include that a choice to 'do nothing' is just as much an active choice as to 'do something', given that both carry the same weight of responsibility for their outcome.

OK, I accept that was two questions really. I don't apologise. The questions stand and it is incumbent on us all to appreciate that we may each be an individual but collectively we carry the short, medium and longer term outcome for the NHS in the conclusions, decisions and actions we engage in. In that, we are all in this together.

A Vital Behavioural Introduction

And here is my first dilemma. At this point you will be dying to hear what I have to say, to see if my rationale has legs, to examine the data and to look for its holes. However, how you react to that rationale is crucial. I'm not trying to influence you but you have to recognise you are already heavily influenced.

Your history, your references, your beliefs, values and even your life plan all have a significant effect on how you interpret what you hear. And it's a problem. To you. I am asking you to look objectively at the facts and circumstances and yet your own biological processing is working against you, even and especially if you are not conscious of it. We have to learn to be better than that. So, that's where I am starting - with a behavioural introduction.

The Danger of Denial

A challenge we all face is to know what's real and what's not. What needs a genuine response and timely action and what's just noise or self-interested persuasion by somebody? How do you know, really? The challenge is made all the more real, complex and difficult to overcome by three confounding factors:

- The greater the challenges, the less we have time to step back, even though that's the very time we should

- It's difficult to assess meaning with no meaningful conceptual framework with which to judge circumstances and new evidence

- The presence of the above two leaves us trying to judge circumstances based on isolated news items or topics, when you need to look at the whole to ascertain authentic meaning

So instead, we judge early, we fill in the gaps, we assume and sometimes we arrive at a meaning that's convenient to us but not necessarily correct though. When faced with tough circumstances, that meaning is frequently a conclusion that things aren't that bad or, for instance, that someone's just going to do something that solves everything. There will be a reality to that question though and it requires objectivity and understanding.

What's clear is that denial is not an adequate strategy because the underlying issues do not go away. In fact, it allows the root causes of our problems to fester and grow. Eventually, the true issues become unignorable but sadly that's too late for many individuals, services and Trusts.

We are seeing those true issues play out in declining performance, job losses, special measures and the imposition of autocratic regulator regimes that ironically tend to exacerbate the very conditions that produced many of the problems in the first place. It could even seem like denial is the default strategy at play in our system. I don't want you to be part of that behavioural trap and certainly not blindly.

To be explicitly clear, denial means it is highly likely you are doing nothing about circumstances that genuinely require something done about them - a meaningful response. If those circumstances have genuine consequences for you as an individual, your service or the Trust as a whole, then you are vulnerable. It's as simple, or complicated, as that.

So, I am going to be unusual. I am going to ask you specifically not to believe a word I say. I am not going to state anything that isn't true or adequately supported by evidence or academia but do not do yourself the injustice of just believing what yet another person says. However, I am going to present a rationale and then ask you to do two things, and even then only if it makes sense as a rationale:

- Firstly, affirm or confirm for yourself what you need to, so that you have confidence in engaging in my next ask

- Secondly, ask yourself what does this mean to you, your services and your Trust and what should you thus do?

If you are worried enough to act but light on insight or suggestions as to what to do and how to do it then at that stage, perhaps I might suggest engaging a little further in discovering some options. However, we are going to start with the rationale and that is about understanding the reality. Options come later. There are options though and it is important to realise some are about survival, some about mitigation and some about emerging stronger in the future.

The Limbic Processing Trap

My last piece of behavioural advice is a piece of education. Whenever we are subject to information or circumstances that are distressing, especially when they might have personal implications, we invoke a deep-seated behavioural reaction that has its foundations in our hunter-gatherer era.

That behavioural reaction is known as a limbic response, generated by our cunningly named limbic system and unfortunately it is designed to produce one totally unhelpful behavioural or cognitive curveball that leads to two frequently unhelpful action responses. Understanding this is key to objectivity and a proper assessment of the likelihood of HealthCRASH. It is also important in acting intelligently i.e. not making matters worse.

Limbic processing is designed to stop you logically and rationally reasoning. That's the unhelpful curveball. Why? Because when you were historically faced with a fierce creature, eyeing you up for dinner, calmly rationalising your circumstances only served to turn you into the very dinner that you were thinking about how to avoid becoming.

So, Mother Nature designed in a fail-safe - bypass the rational thinking in favour of a near-instant, emotionally-driven fight or flight response - the two unhelpful outputs. Biologically, we really struggle to separate physical threat from career threat, organisational risk, financial threat etc. Why? Because even the separation process requires thinking - the one commodity you are robbed of really early on in this behavioural process.

Consequently, courtesy of Mother Nature and with not an insignificant amount of additional help by healthcare policy makers, movers and shakers, we have 1.3 million healthcare people in a melting pot of risky and threatening circumstances, all struggling to really think things through and know what to do for the best.

Instead they are reacting, emotionally, in ways that mostly are not in their own best interests, or in the best interests of their services, organisations and the NHS as a whole but to which they are rendered cognitively blind by the very mental system that purports to be about saving them. Blind - yes, they don't even know it. In case it escaped your notice, you are almost certainly 1 of those 1.3 million cognitively blind individuals.

I am guessing though that if you are reading still, you might be at least somewhat worried you could be one of them and that's OK. Not only does it make you human but you have also started in down the track of greater clarity by developing some self-awareness. I have also tried to take this into account as I unfold this rationale, although being human myself there is always the possibility I haven't got it quite perfect just yet.

If you'd like a small tool or technique that might help, try the following. Whenever you have an emotion or reaction about something, ask yourself these three questions:

- What am I thinking that is giving rise to these feelings?

- Do those thoughts have any basis in fact or evidence?

- If not, what other thoughts or meanings are at least possible?

13

The process of asking these questions is to force your brain back out of limbic mode and on to examining other possibilities, not to mention exposing the assumptions and flaws in your own thinking. With that in mind, let's start examining the rationale for HealthCRASH. To do that, we need an adequate and objective conceptual framework.

Analysing our Circumstances

The next challenge we face is just how to go about analysing something as complicated as how our system works and whether it is likely to stop working any time soon. This is not an insignificant issue because to fully appreciate whether or not we are entering HealthCRASH, we need to bring together a wide range of factors but make sense of them together.

As you have probably discovered, it is difficult enough to understand how a system as complex as healthcare really works, let alone how that might change if we shift a few parameters. That becomes all the more difficult when the very system itself is in flux. We are presented with dilemmas such as whether the system is changing because of circumstances or whether the circumstances are a function of a changing system. Or both.

For instance, do we have austerity in the provider sector because of changes to the tariff system and commissioning, or are we subject to tariff changes and commissioning initiatives because we have failed to fix austerity or sustainability? You can see that how we interpret that question not only might influence whether we see austerity as the problem or someone's partial solution to their resultant problem but also could be utilised to justify one of two diametrically opposite policy positions!

I am going to suggest that to adequately understand what's happening and what it means to us, we need a conceptual framework. We need a way of looking at the problem or question I am proposing - whether our NHS is entering what I describe as HealthCRASH.

Simple Conceptual Framework

At severe risk of appearing to trivialise something that is anything but trivial, I am going to conceptualise our current crisis (and I don't think there's much debate whether we are in one of those but CRASH is a different ball game) with a POOP analogy. It goes like this and it is surprisingly useful in thinking through the issues:

For us to be irreversible in the poop (I know, you thought it was an acronym but I did say analogy) i.e. in HealthCRASH, four primary conditions have to be met:

1. There has to be something generating a level of poop that we can't just get out of easily and certainly not in a timescale consistent with survival, and...

2. We do actually have to be genuinely in the poop i.e. we are being adversely affected by it, and...

3. We would need to be rendered sufficiently helpless that our best efforts would not get us out of the poop in time to save us, and, finally...

4. There is no likely prospect of being rescued from the poop by anybody else e.g. Government in our case

You could also say that being in the poop would need to matter to individuals, services and Trusts or it would render the other four conditions pointless. I am guessing you are reading because it matters to you, unless you have a very funny idea of light entertainment.

Sadly though, there is a significant element or piece of denial that's been long running and learned through a history of organisational failure and subsequent rescue by the system. It does result in the misplaced belief that being in the poop in an organisation doesn't actually matter i.e. have individual consequences. However, that long-run assumption will be addressed and crushed when we come to examine condition 4 above, which I will explain in due course.

To turn that simple conceptual framework into our healthcare reality, I am asking you to answer four questions, based on logic, rational reasoning, evidence and data:

- Are the challenges affecting our society and health system sufficiently large to crash that system or render it unsustainable?
- If so, can we see genuine evidence of system decline as a direction of travel?
- Do we have the capability to find a solution and then lead a level of transformation sufficiently swiftly that it genuinely saves the healthcare system?
- And if it's a "yes, yes, no" to those, is there a real prospect or likelihood that Government can or will rescue the healthcare system (and if not them, whom)?

These are tough questions with complex answers that too few are looking at. Furthermore, many of those who are looking, are looking in simplistic ways, underpinned by out-dated assumptions and often without using the facts and evidence. That's very scary and wholly unjust. Lives and livelihoods depend on our NHS. It, patients and we all deserve more.

However, to convey all of this in a single sitting is a big ask, especially given the low reading tolerance we have in our over-busy lives. So, I am approaching it in two phases - a very detailed 'outline' or narrative that if sufficiently compelling will encourage you to examine the true detail in greater depth. I can do no more.

A Final Word of Caution & Reassurance

This narrative is focused on the rather singular issue of whether HealthCRASH is a distinct possibility or likelihood. If you start to conclude that it is, you will find a weird little mental process starting up that becomes rather uncomfortable and destructive. It's again a limbic-type response and again it has the potential to leave us inadvertently vulnerable. Let's take a quick look and then on with real work, mentally prepared and on guard.

The more you start to conclude that HealthCRASH is a likelihood, the more you'll start to 'want' that not to be the case. Why? Because it means something that is really quite unpleasant and possibly threatening. Our first line of defence is frequently to 'hope' that it isn't real and seek evidence to validate that hope. Yes, it's a form of denial.

Ironically, your true individual vulnerability lies in failing to act meaningfully or intelligently when the threat is genuinely real. The above little process unfortunately leads into that very trap. It can be heightened when you don't have solutions or know what to do and hence my raising it now, before you fall into it.

If, and I have been openly forthright in reinforcing IF, you genuinely feel that the possibility is real, then we can look at the sorts of things you can do to mitigate the effects of HealthCRASH, at an individual, service and Trust level. HealthCRASH at a system-level will require individuals, services and Trusts to do specific things to mitigate its effects.

I am really saying let's first decide on the possibility and THEN we'll look at the options. At this stage, I just want to reassure you that there are options and indeed opportunities. HealthCRASH will be catastrophic for many, highly scary and unpleasant for most but also highly beneficial for some - the ready, the prepared and the adaptable.

As you can probably gather, it's those that learn to address or compensate for those feelings, develop a deeper, clearer understanding and then determine a sensible and appropriate course of action that tend to fare best. The research is pretty clear that's about 20% left to their own devices, the remaining 80% developing a less than optimal to downright maladaptive set of responses. The biggest challenge? The 80% believe they are in the 20%!

How We'll Examine HealthCRASH Likelihood

I am going to work through this in the order of the four questions. However, to fully understand, we have to appreciate that they are interrelated. We can exacerbate crisis severity by the actions we take, which is linked to our capability to find meaningful solutions, or not. A group with every capability could make poor choices and precipitate a disaster.

To reiterate this and to start into our analysis with a clear mind, the four questions are:

- Q1. Are the challenges affecting our society and health system sufficiently large to crash that system or render it unsustainable?
- Q2. If so, can we see genuine evidence of system decline as a direction of travel?
- Q3. Do we have the capability to find a solution and then lead a level of transformation sufficiently swiftly that it genuinely saves the healthcare system?
- Q4. And if it's a "yes, yes, no" to those, is there a real prospect or likelihood that Government can or will rescue the healthcare system (and if not them, whom)?

All four questions needs to be satisfied appropriately for HealthCRASH to be a likelihood. I don't want to over-conclude any more than I want to under-conclude.

There are few absolutes and a myriad of variations. I am approaching this 'on balance' and trying to take into account the general position we find ourselves in. For instance, you could be part of a highly successful Trust surrounded by other Trusts spiralling out of control. For all your best efforts, capability and starting point, it is easy to find their actions become your unresolvable problems. We have to consider all aspects to stand the best chance of a reasonable conclusion one way or the other.

Q1. Are the Challenges Big Enough

In this, I don't think many would question the severity of the issues we face. We have a growing crisis, precipitated by a multitude of factors with population and economics at the heart of it. However, despite that acceptance of the problem, I do think the overall depth of understanding in the specifics is low and that leads us to not even asking whether it is big enough to cause HealthCRASH.

Why do I think too few understand in depth? Because the response to the crisis is wholly inadequate to the magnitude (more on this later) and this suggests either that too few people understand it or that they can't relate what it really means. Either way, it's easy to overlook the true meaning if you don't know the specifics.

To simplify, the crisis we face has 4 core components, any one of which would be difficult to contend with. However, it's the convergence of the 4 that creates such a magnitude of crisis and certainly a magnitude sufficient to produce HealthCRASH. By way of a teeny bit of writing indulgence, I am going to refer to these as the 4 Horseman of the Healthcare Apocalypse!

Population

Over the next 20 years or so, we are going to see a 17% growth in the population overall but a near doubling of the population age bands that already consume nearly 50% of all healthcare resources. If you nearly double the group that consumes nearly half, that's a near 50% increase in demand over that period, without the effects of the other Horsemen. If you don't know these figures and what they really mean, intimately, then you need to because they go to the heart of developing a response of the right magnitude and nature.

We need to consider this for its implications not its headlines. Population is increasing across all age bands but by far the fastest in the older age bands. Data from the Office of National Statistics (ONS) illustrates that our primary tax paying bands collectively will rise by just 7.7% over the next 20 - 25 years. However, our highest healthcare demand group, the over 75 age band, will rise by 81.8% in the same period. Even within that upper band, it's the over 85 age group that is increasing the fastest.

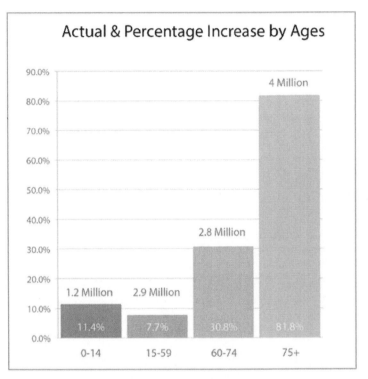

Figure 1. Actual and Percentage Increases in Population by Age Band (using data from the ONS)

Importantly, when considering the implications of this, we need to consider that the greatest impacts will likely be borne by the least well equipped and sustainable part of our system - social care. If we are struggling with social care presently (and I don't think anybody would argue whether we are), imagine the issues we will face when there are twice as many individuals for them to cope with, in an era of reducing resource (which we'll come back to later).

By way of further explanation but without wanting to overwhelm you, our population increases in the way that it does of the interplay between three figures or rates; the birth rate, the death rate and the net migration rate. Although net migration has risen in recent years, the difference between the birth rate and death rate is the predominant influence and what causes a demographic shift in age balance.

Figure 2 shows that in the 1960s we had a very high birth-rate and a big gap between this and the death rate. That has become known as the baby-boomer period for obvious reasons. Those baby-boomers are now getting older and it is this 'glut' of people living ever longer that is driving an ageing population.

UK Debt Interest Payments

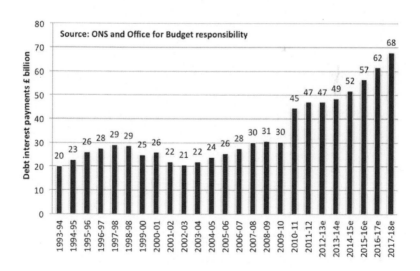

Figure 2. ONS Birth-rate & Death-rate Curves

You can clearly see that we have a big gap today and how impactful the falling death rate is. To be clear, the reason we have fewer deaths is an increasing life expectancy. The death rate above is not the 'likelihood' of dying but the actual number of deaths, which is itself a function of the population size at different age bands AND the likelihood of dying at each of them too.

There are two arguments that you will hear against the likelihood of HealthCRASH. The first is that excessive healthcare spend or consumption is largely devoted to the last year of life and the second is that this is a problem that reverts over time. Dealing with the second first, this is true. However, it absolutely does not revert in a timescale that prevents HealthCRASH, given that we get peak effect over the next 20 years or so.

The second argument (first above) is more complex and I am only going to deal with part of it now. That is simply to say that regardless of how right or wrong this assumption is, we are going to have a lot more last years of life over the coming years!

Sources of Population Data

Without question, the singular most reliable source of population data and predictions is the Office of national Statistics. It is their figures I have used in this narrative. For further information, I suggest a visit to the population section of their website at:

http://ons.gov.uk/ons/taxonomy/index.html?nscl=Population

Economics

I am sure you are not immune to the headlines that we apparently have a strong economy when compared to our western neighbours. However, it depends on how you describe 'strong' though.

I have spent a huge length of time examining our economics in great depth from multiple sources but then I am interested in it. However, I am conscious that if I write here in a level of detail matched to my enthusiasm for the topic, you might not get past this section. You do need to know the basics though. For those that really like to check facts and details, or who share my interest, I have included a much bigger 'sources' section at the end of this synthesis. So here goes...

We have a 'stronger' rate of growth than some of our western neighbours but it is largely debt-fuelled. That has consequences, not least of which is a question over how real that growth really is and how sustainable it is likely to be, especially if and when we can no longer rely on debt.

It also goes to the heart of policy differences between say Mr Osbourne (a proponent of austerity and living within our economic means) and Mr Corbyn (perhaps as politically opposite as you could get, having been elected to position leadership on an anti-austerity vote). This is important when we start to consider what Governments are able to do and what they have the propensity to do, a vital consideration later when we examine potential rescuers.

Let's examine debt. Debt interest is our 4th largest area of national spend (we spend about 50% more on debt interest than we do on defence, just to put it in context) and we run a year-on-year budget deficit that is larger (as a proportion of GDP) than ANY other country on the planet, including being worse than Spain, Italy, Portugal or Greece. That is not a healthy position, quite the opposite.

We have to consider two things. That debt interest continues to climb at an accelerating rate and debt as a whole continues to climb, despite the height of austerity. In the 2014/15 financial year, Britain had a budget deficit of £87.3 billion, which effectively is additional borrowing. This deficit is greater than any other EU country.

UK Debt Interest Payments

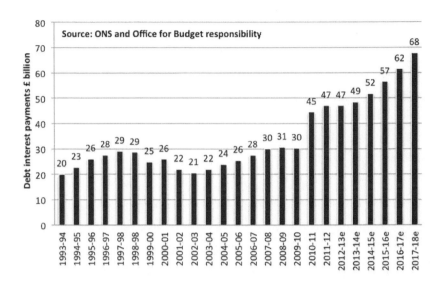

Figure 3. UK Debt Interest. Actual & Projections

Our actual Government debt stands at £1.56 trillion as of end of quarter 1 in 2015. As you can see from Figure 4, that has risen exponentially from the early-1970s, after being low for most of the previous century. Whereas we must consider that our economic ability to service that debt has also grown, it should be clear to all that it has not followed the same trajectory (or we wouldn't be debating HealthCRASH!).

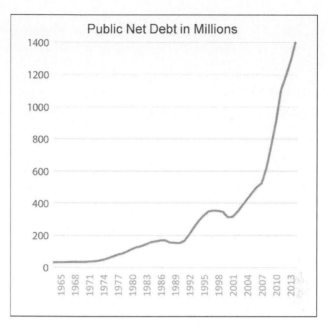

Figure 4. Public Net Debt in Millions (ONS Data)

So what has allowed debt to swell that much? This is essentially an interest rate phenomenon, coupled to growth in economic output. It is best to think of this as a person and the debt as loans and credit cards. Each year the person earns little more (very little more, if you are public sector at the present time!). And, over time since the 1970s, the cost of borrowing i.e. interest rate, has dropped down to its current historic low (it has never been this low since the Bank of England starts collecting the data in 1694), it's long run average being around 5%.

This has allowed Bob, our pseudonym for a rather fiscally irresponsible 'person' (Government) to take out more debt each year because it is slightly more affordable and Bob has slightly more earnings. He now finds himself with this monumental level of debt, only made possible because interest rates kept falling to their present near zero level. And now Bob finds himself in a rather uncomfortable position in that his salary increases (economic growth) have slowed down and his interest rates are unlikely to stay so low over time. He is stuck. He can't afford for rates to rise, which is why, I suspect, that the Bank of England has found good reason not to each time they said they would.

Some may argue that we have historically had higher levels of debt when measured as a percentage of economic output (GDP). However, that was predominantly immediately post world wars when we carried huge excess debts on very low economic output. We didn't so much pay that off as deflate it i.e. high inflation reduces its net value year-on-year. That's just as uncomfortable for us because we have negative inflation at the time of writing and a sharp rise is unlikely (and unwelcome on our household spending).

So, here we are. Our annual income as a country falls considerably short of our expenditure already and economic growth is not closing that gap. Economists predict that economic growth in western nations will remain chronically low for decades, presenting western Governments and ours in particular with a monumental problem - an economy based on a higher rate of growth, already deeply in the red annually, with enormous levels of debt and little prospect of any significant near-term reversion.

None of this is supposition or speculation. The deficit, debt, growth and economic analyses are available to all that choose to look. They explain a majority of recent, apparently strange, Government decisions, when you realise, plain and simple, that the Government just doesn't have access to sufficient money (taxation or borrowing - their two main sources) to maintain current national infrastructure such as healthcare.

To explain that further, when ministers appear to be in denial over how much something genuinely costs, we need to consider that their decisions are more likely to be based on full knowledge but no meaningful options, denial therefore feeling like the easiest solution. We tend to view Government as blind, detached and inept and yet it is full of highly intelligent people, supported by even more intelligent people, all armed with immensely granular data. But, if you have no cash, you have no cash.

What does this real mean for us and our analysis of the potential for HealthCRASH? Government just does not have the money to cover the true underlying cost of providing healthcare, today, let alone tomorrow and we have seen this in their failure to keep track with costs, a recent year-on-year reduction across many tariffs as part of CIP and the addition of marginal rates, latterly in specialist care, an area of care that just does not lend itself to economies of scale.

There is a myriad of figures I could present to support these conclusions and they are all laid out clearly in some of the programmes I deliver to clinical and non-clinical groups, such as our Insights Programme. It's a very unpalatable prospect to consider we are dependent on a Government that is devoid of the necessary cash but which refuses to be open about that predicament.

I am also guessing that there is the potential as this moment for you to be thinking "surely that can't really be the case", as you start to rely on that 'wish it was different' sense of hope. However, if that 'denial' is creeping in, it's a good moment for me to ask if you actually know the figures i.e. are basing your 'hope' conclusion on real data, comprehensively examined and approached without emotional bias? I'm asking for nothing more than that. If you don't know the data, go look.

Once you have satisfied yourself of the validity of the arguments, you'll be left with a foreboding sense that what you were 'hoping' might happen (Government suddenly saying "oh yes, we just need to provide more money") could just be impossible, or certainly very, very difficult and not without pain in others areas.

Sources of Economic Information

There are a multitude of these and I will point you towards what I think are the most pertinent and accessible.

Office of national Statistics. Go to the section on the economy, although useful data is elsewhere too.

http://ons.gov.uk/ons/taxonomy/index.html?nscl=Economy

Trading Economics. Simply select the country in question.

http://www.tradingeconomics.com/

Capital Economics. Good for predictions and prospects, from the incredible intelligent and frighteningly accurate in prediction Roger Bootle, adviser to Governments etc.

https://www.capitaleconomics.com/

Economics Help. A good place to start for basic things and lots of graphs & tables.

http://www.economicshelp.org/

Office for Budget Responsibility. The Government's own department for transparency (yes, I recognise the hypocrisy), good for national budgets and expenditure but you can check them against ONS data too!

http://budgetresponsibility.org.uk/

The Spectator. Used as antidote to the hypocrisy and misleading engaged in by Government, as they are really quite good at pointing out ministers who say one thing when the data says another.

http://blogs.new.spectator.co.uk/category/coffeehouse/

Care Complexity

With an ageing population comes an increase in healthcare complexity. We saw the effects of this in winter 2014/15 when comparatively small increases in attendances and admissions totally overwhelmed A&E and hospitals in general, resulting in a near cessation of elective work and even tents in carparks for some. A number of Trusts declared major emergencies.

At the time, people felt it as an onslaught. Post-event, Monitor undertook a detailed analysis of the circumstances and determined that although numbers were up somewhat, in no way did it explain the severity of the circumstances. What did, however, was the clear finding about increased acuity and complexity - patients required more work on average and so a small increase in numbers produced an exponential rise in healthcare input required. I am guessing that I don't have to persuade you of this because you experienced it for yourself.

There is an important question though, with a less clear answer about why A&E ended up with these patients in higher numbers (an ongoing debate, of course) but that is more than adequately explained by the strain on social care, increasing the chances of an individual developing an acute episode. Ironically, a reduction in social care inputs is likely to have a disproportionately adverse effect on secondary care load because it will most likely be the sicker, more complex individuals that end up with an episode severe enough to send them to hospital.

As population increases and ages, these are issues that are only going to get worse, despite services being at breaking point already. Social care is in real trouble and that has a significant knock-on effect for the NHS. Dementia adds to this issue tremendously by turning a straight-forward patient into a complex one. Nothing has happened between last winter and this one to alleviate that problem and we should probably be battening down the hatches in preparation for an even bigger storm.

As a more general challenge, it also doesn't help that our systems have not been designed around the very specific needs of certain high-consumption groups of patients that we have today, although that's a domain where we could also make real gains. As an example, my own Mother-in-Law, with dementia, ended up with a 21 day stay for radiological assessments. Not only did she occupy an otherwise needed surgical bed, as a way of undertaking her diagnosis, it was completely at odds with her background needs as a complex patient. It occurred because of both pressure and poor design issues.

Reforming the ways services are delivered is a crux of central policy and part of Mr Stevens answer to reducing the gap between cost of demand and available funding. However, transforming services and care to match up to the needs of a few high-consumption patients instead of the many, is a complex behavioural challenge in its own right and one with a very chequered history of success (or failure, more commonly).

The truth is that we base our funding, projections and capacity on the changing numbers of patients, not the increased complexity. However, if you increase the numbers and the complexity concurrently, you see an exponential increase in demand, not linear. Simply, each patient takes more work and stays longer, on average. When we add the increasing numbers effect, to the increasing complexity effect and the poor economics effect, you are starting to get a picture of a challenge that is gargantuan and almost certainly unresolvable, however unpalatable and difficult to comprehend that may be.

However, if that is a reality considered by Government (and it is even more scary to think that they might not have), it would go a long way to explain so many of the policies, constraints and changes they have made that just do not make sense when looked at through any other lens.

Daily, I am asked "doesn't the Government 'know' what their policies are doing and how much destruction they are causing?"

from people who see something like a hospital going into administration as an unpalatable consequence of poor central decisions and actions. I would assert that they know exactly what is happening and 'accept' it as a natural consequence of circumstances that at best are only partially resolvable in their eyes and thus also warrant a set of policies that are as much about damage limitation and political protection (think devolution, lead provider etc).

Advances

Ironically, it is our ability to innovate in clinical care that in part has produced the magnitude of problem we have today. Year-on-year there is more that we can do for a patient and the growth of open communication through the media and social media means that patients know this. Not only does this result in significantly increased healthcare costs per patient, it creates the single biggest demand influence - the gradual shift of life-threatening diseases towards chronic diseases.

A disease with a significant mortality is like a bucket with a hole. Every year we find more patients and every year we lose some too. The disease burden is relatively static. However, partially solve that disease through medical advance and you fill in the hole in the bucket but without turning off the tap that's filling it. The bucket fills up very rapidly and those now surviving patients go on to get other nasty, expensive stuff too. The shift in life-expectancy in diabetes alone has created a diabetes population of 3 million with a life expectancy that even allows them to suffer from dementia! That's a huge shift in disease burden.

We need to be clear why this effect is so great and diabetes is a great example. When the NHS formed in 1948 there was comparatively little diabetes and what there was had a relatively low life expectancy. Since then, we have seen the emergency of huge populations with type 2 diabetes but those patients now have a life expectancy only 6 years shorter than normal. When we are thinking about the impact on healthcare demand, we have to consider:

- The cost of diabetes care for 3+ million people

- The cost of complications of diabetes (heart disease, amputations, eye problems etc)

- The cost of care for complaints they otherwise wouldn't have got e.g. dementia, older age cancers etc

When considered in this fashion, we can see that although diabetes care is a true medical success story that has positively changed the life course for so many, it has come with an exponentially increasing disease burden cost and one that the NHS was never designed to cope with. And we aren't coping very well.

Furthermore, in 1948 we set up an acute disease treatment service and these advances in medical science leave us predominantly with a chronic disease management burden. Whereas many acute diseases lend themselves most appropriately to hospital-based care, chronic diseases really require a different model, especially for ageing, increasingly frail individuals how might have difficulties like dementia too.

We haven't fundamentally changed the shape of our system very much and the question now is, just how do you do that when you haven't got enough money. The answer is re-distribute within the NHS ring-fence, which we are seeing much more. The predicament this creates is the time lag, resulting in secondary care having funding removed whilst they are still providing the care, itself contributing to the likelihood of HealthCRASH.

Diabetes is not the only condition that fits this profile. The answer is clearly to simultaneously work towards an outright cure whilst also massively increasing our research and approaches to reducing the numbers of new patients (working on the tap end of the equation). However, we have to accept that this research takes decades and that the pharmaceutical industry favours research into treatments rather than preventions, for obvious commercial reasons. Furthermore, we have just seen a reduction in the budget for public health, itself telling about what the Government thinks about this as a course of action and whether its benefit arrives in time to save the day.

In Summary of our 4 Horsemen

So that concludes my look at and narrative about the sheer magnitude of the bigger picture issues that are collectively poop-producing towards HealthCRASH. It also helps start to explain some of the policy decisions and indeed in-decisions we are seeing.

I have tried to convey a sense of the magnitude of the challenges we face as a country, in relation to sustaining a healthcare service of the type and funding model we are used to. Any one of these 4 domains creates a near-insurmountable challenge. However, it is the combination of the four, all converging and peaking in the same 20 year timespan that creates a tsunami-strength tidal wave that probably leaves you and must leave Government somewhat with a sense of futility. The question is whether this magnitude is sufficient to precipitate HealthCRASH. I would ask you to draw your own conclusions.

The magnitude of the challenge is not the only consideration though, even though it feels like facing-down that tsunami armed with something that now looks a bit like a wicker fence, rather than sea defences. It is what we can and are able to do about it that is the equally important discussion we must now turn to.

When we are considering the question of HealthCRASH, we have to consider speed of that tidal wave, not just its magnitude. Conceptually, we could build incredible sea-defences but ONLY if we have the money and ONLY if we have the time and even then ONLY if we have the capability. Lastly, we have to recognise just how difficult it is to build those sea defences if we are already under water and that is question 2 on our list.

Q2. Evidence of a System in Decline

In the interests of objectivity, I don't want to short cut a section that many will take as a given. Equally, there are some distinctions to be made about the severity of meaning of evidence in different domains. My early assertion is that the NHS as a whole conveniently ignores or denies some of the most impactful areas, such as staff morale. Evidence is crucial and again we have to consider it together, not in isolated pieces. You can conceive of all the hypotheses in the world but if they aren't exhibiting themselves in real life then you have to reconsider those hypotheses.

Additionally, we are considering the possibility of HealthCRASH, a hypothesis with huge implications for individuals, services and Trusts, not to mention patients and the public at large. There's a huge difference between evidence of 'the odd difficulty' and that which suggests a fairly catastrophic slide. We would want to see sufficient evidence of sufficient severity. Ironically, said evidence arrived today, prior to me getting to this very point in the rationale. And that's where we will start.

Financial Decline

In quarter 1 of the 2015/16 financial year, the 241 Trusts reported on by Monitor (Foundation Trusts) and the Trust Development Authority (TDA - for Non-Foundation Trusts) amassed a combined deficit of £930 million, putting 79% of them in the deficit category and greater than 80% of the acute sector specifically. That needs putting in context. Last year, the combined deficit across all providers was £822 million at year end i.e. the quarter 1 deficit this year is greater than the total deficit for last year.

Earlier this year, when the figures were assembled, checked and finalised for last year, NHS England (NHSE) and Mr Hunt were both saying that providers needed to get a grip and that a result like this was unacceptable and unsustainable. At that time, Trusts were also asked for their 2015/16 forecasts and the aggregate deficit at that point was £2.1 billion. Now that was a figure to cause palpitations in many and shockwaves higher up the system and into Government.

The reaction to this by the Department of Health (DH), NHSE and Jeremy Hunt was swift - this was unacceptable, fundamentally unaffordable and it had to change.

Monitor were dispatched to the 43 Foundation Trusts (FTs) predicting the biggest deficits to forensically go through their books and encourage reductions. At the same time, the TDA were tasked with leading 'stretch targets' into their non-FTs, typically around £3 - £5 million on a Trust deficit of around £17 million, as an example. It is important to know and reflect on that neither approach to deficit reduction involved any kind of meaningful solution and those of you that have participated in those meetings or phone calls will know only too well that the rhetoric was "fix it, or else".

How serious this decline was already at that stage should have been noted when a number of Trusts came out in the media and said "we'll take 'or else' because there just isn't any more blood in the already bone dry stone and we're not prepared to harm patient care". Worryingly, some said "OK, we'll get to it" and consequently I suspect there is a looming set of clinical issues lurking below the surface and that is something we have all feared for some time now. This won't have helped one bit.

Further evidence of the systematic financial decline of the system comes from the changes made to how struggling Trusts are supported. These changes and evidence are significant because they point to a whole system running out of options and engaging in some poor financial practise as a result.

The first was to start raiding capital reserves, a move I liken to selling off the family silver. The point is, once it's gone it's gone. It's a last resort. The second change was to switch from providing various forms of operational support to loans. And that's tantamount to a scandal that these latest results expose.

Operational support is highly visible from an accounting perspective because it is treated as a cost. However, a loan is not treated as a cost. In fact, it can be treated as an asset, exactly the issue that gave rise to the greatest scandal of this type - the banking crisis. In said crisis, parent organisations (banks) lent money to individuals in amounts that couldn't realistically be paid back. They then accounted for those loans as assets, giving the illusion of bank financial health, when in fact those loans stood no chance of repayment, resulting in the collapse of the banking system. I would be shocked if you haven't picked up on the identical nature of this behaviour. Of course, we threw the perpetrators of the banking crisis out of jobs and even in jail. Sadly, we just re-elected our NHS-crisis perpetrators.

If you need further evidence about how serious this is, consider that this latest data, pointing to a near £4 billion deficit across the year, is actually very late. Monitor's announcement specifically points to it being prepared for the 30th September NHSE Board Meeting. Without wanting to speculate who, how or why, it has appeared only now, just after the end of the Tory Party Conference. Given my earlier warnings about denial, this represents denial on a gargantuan scale, with a big dose of collusion to go with it. That's FACT, not conspiracy or speculation.

It's also not the only behaviour of its kind and we are seeing that 'type' of behaviour creep in with greater regularity. Delaying or manipulating the release of negative financial news is in part a classic example of denial. The problem hasn't gone away or even changed in form. So why not be honest and open.

Another recent financially-driven example was the cancellation of the body of work that The National Institute for Health and Care Excellence (NICE) had been conducting around safe staffing levels, itself a response to clinical decline at the hands of cost reduction activity, in favour of bringing the work 'in house' inside DH. In direct response to that cancellation, NICE, a legally independent organisation, took the decision that they would publish their work anyway, also suggesting that officials shouldn't commission work or ask questions if they aren't prepared for the reality of the answers.

To be clear, suppression of guidance because it is financially uncomfortable is evidence of denial at a senior level AND of financial decline in the system, or those same people wouldn't be so worried. The safe staffing work was a recommendation of Lord Francis in response to the Mid Staffordshire crisis and he immediately expressed serious concerns about its suspension. As if to confirm that, the suspension of safe staffing guidance for A&E staff was widely reported as being due to concerns over soaring agency fees. It was a financial driver, not a safety one that caused the suspension.

As if the story could get worse, NICE did not publish its safe staffing guidance after all, but why? It would appear that the direct cause of this was more political leaning by Mr Hunt's office and it was the NICE Chief Executive, Sir Andrew Dhillon, that was lent on. Far from conspiracy, this was reported in Health Service Journal on 14th October 2015, who also took the trouble to release the correspondence into the public domain. But what does this all mean?

We are seeing a level of actual financial decline that is producing a whole host of what can only be described as panic behaviours in senior places. These include suppression of data, safety policies abandoned for financial reasons, political influence or leaning and a raft of ill-thought-through, poorly aligned policies, initiatives and behaviours that are direct functions of that panic.

That there is such a level of panic in such high places, the people we pay top dollar for in the hope that they'll remain calm in a crisis and act intelligently, is clear evidence of the decline already present. Add to that the catastrophic 2015 quarter 1 figures and the deeply uncomfortable realisation that the figures are all going in the wrong direction despite ALL of the initiatives and policies, and you have fairly unequivocal evidence of a level of financial decline that is enough to precipitate HealthCRASH by creating an almost impossible to recover from deficit. And that's before we look at functional decline.

Operational Decline

Alongside the accelerating decline in financial health, we are starting to see the true effects of the wrong type of cost-saving measures in a system that was already bone dry. Across virtually EVERY performance measure that covers operational delivery effectiveness, we are seeing a system-wide decline. The consistency is as telling as the magnitude. We aren't just struggling in some areas, we are struggling in virtually ALL areas and this is despite the level of work being applied to some to regain target adherence.

Accident & Emergency

At the time of writing, the FT sector had failed to meet the 4-hour waiting time target for a 6th successive quarter. The first quarter 2015/16 performance of 94.5% was a year-on-year reduction from 2014/15. Monitor were quick to point out that it was a significant improvement on the previous quarter but when we consider that the previous quarter came in below 92%, a level not seen since the targets were first introduced i.e. before we had ever attained a target in A&E, that is really a paltry consolation.

Without regurgitating the reasons, they do link back to some of our bigger picture population shifts with increased admissions through major A&E (Type 1) departments and a more complex case mix both being at play. If that is affecting healthcare, we'd expect it to be affecting social care even more and there's a very real concern that failing to look after and support frail individuals allows them to become some of our most complex, admitted secondary care patients, often through A&E.

The confirming data comes from the very same Monitor report, indicating that the number of bed days lost to Delayed Transfers of Care (DToCs) had risen to 73,500 in the quarter, a 5.5% increase on the same quarter in previous years. To fully appreciate the pressure this causes, we need to consider the ramifications of a complex problem that includes:

- More patients
- Sicker, more complex patients
- Fewer acute beds
- DToCs

Those ramifications at the patient end meant an increase in over four-hour trolley waits from 21,700 in Q1 for 2014/15 to 29,500 in Q1 this year. Let's be clear, that's a 35.9% increase in a year, perhaps indicating that even a small challenge to our at capacity, overwhelmed, on the edge system produces quite a significant level of operational failure and sometimes with some very unpleasant consequences for patients.

Elective Treatment

The very helpful analyses by Rob Findlay from Gooroo, highlight the largest ever year-on-year August increase in patients waiting more than 18 weeks for the commencement of their hospital elective care. In fact, of the major surgical specialties, only gynaecology, ophthalmology and ENT are still achieving the 18 week target. Furthermore, all of the gains seen in the run up to the May 2015 election have been lost, demonstrating that you can buy better figures if you are in charge of the allocation but the underlying reality is a decline.

There is an unseen financial story in the background of this operational decline. Given the marginal rates attached to emergency care, this slide in operational delivery of elective care is particularly serious because it heralds a shift in balance between emergency and elective resulting usually from insufficient capacity to handle both. The net effect is to reduce income without reducing costs, thus increasing the deficit many Trusts have. We have to recognise the vicious circle in this.

Following Bruce Keogh's review of waiting time standards, NHS England formally removed both admitted and non-admitted referral to treatment (RTT) standards in June of this year, 2015. The RTT incomplete standard has now become the sole measure of waiting time performance. Whether this is prompted by a desire to simplify the reporting requirements or a fear of what the more granular targets might show we will probably never know. However, declines in RTT do need to be understood for their implications.

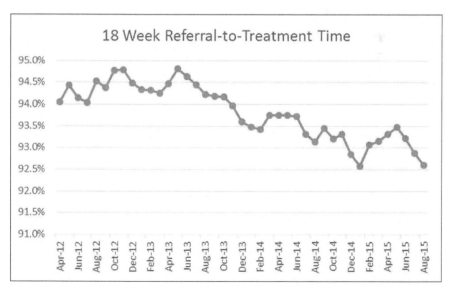

Figure 5. Percentage of Patients seen within 18 Weeks. Source NHS England.

Figure 5 shows a near-linear reduction in the percentage of patients seen within 18 weeks over the last 2 years, with the greatest declines seen in the difficult winter periods, followed by some recovery in subsequent quarters. However, the recent August data shows an alarming rate of decline.

The most immediate and visible impact of decline is on the number of patients waiting more than 18 weeks, shown in Figure 6. That the number appears to be accelerating is of concern for a number of reasons, some of which go to the heart of individual provider vulnerability and others perhaps contributing to higher A&E demand. At a system level, it is saying that more and more patients are finding the NHS isn't there for them at the point of need.

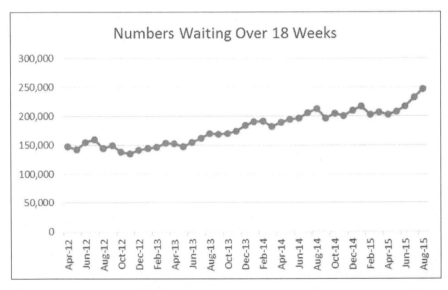

Figure 6. Number of Patients Waiting Over 18 Weeks. Source NHS England.

Some would argue that an elderly lady waiting a few more weeks for a knee replacement is hardly a clinical catastrophe.

However, it might be a social one. Her reduced mobility may well contribute to a further loss of functional stability that she may not get back with considerable support, support that increasingly is not available. She may have a higher risk of a fall, on stairs for instance. It may contribute to an increase in social care requirements or demands, many of which are not adequately met. At the very least, it will create, as an average, a higher degree of complexity or severity and that is likely to lead to longer lengths of stay and a greater need for formal rehabilitation, which will increase the likelihood of more DToCs and so the spiral continues.

Moreover, a growing number of patients waiting longer and longer creates a very real business risk for Trusts. In an era of patient choice and the growth of private providers holding NHS provider licenses e.g. BUPA, Shire and others, long access times increase the risk that a patient will book with another provider, redistributing the funding. That is likely to precipitate a commissioner-led re-balancing of the local contracts for that elective care, resulting in the original provider having a lower threshold number of cases to cross before going onto a marginal (lower) rate per case. It is also possible that persisting or worsening long access times opens up the region to the entrance of a new provider e.g. Circle Health. This again causes contract dilution and weakens the position of the existing provider.

The key point is that we have markedly declining performance in elective access times and that is both evidence of significant operational decline AND increased provider vulnerability. It is almost certainly at least a contributing factor in worsening A&E performance and in-patient burden. We are dangerously close to losing attainment of the 18 week RTT target, presenting a whole new problem too - that patients have a legal right to treatment within 18 weeks. We have to ask how that might be fulfilled if the providers can't do it.

We are seeing an uncomfortable rate of decline in attainment of the cancer referral to treatment time targets, illustrated clearly in Figure 7. That rate of decline has been steep and linear for two whole years.

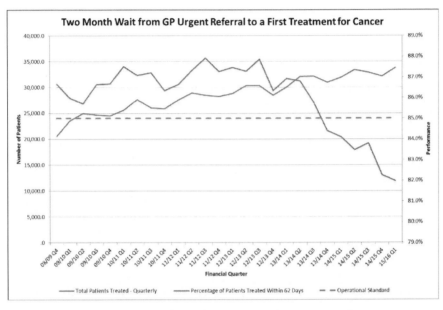

Figure 7. 62-day Referral to First Treatment for Cancer Performance.
Source NHS England.

Figure 7 tells us another story about our circumstances too. Although the number of referrals has been increasing, not surprising with an increasing and ageing population, that increase is fairly linear and comparatively low. However, the rate of decline in attainment of the 62-day target is steep. What this suggests is a system over the edge of capacity, so that any additional load has a disproportionately adverse effect on performance.

This is something we should take notice of because we can already conclude that in something as emotive and important as cancer, we already have a system evidencing significant and rapid decline. But worryingly, although far from unexpectedly, demand continues to rise, itself taking a breaking system and breaking it still further. We have to reflect that this comes at a time when providers are being asked to spend less and not use agency staff, making it very difficult to add back in what is almost certainly a necessary increase in capacity.

To pour further fuel on that fire, we may well need more professionals that just don't exist as the system as a whole adopts a reductionist set of policies across the board, without really considering the differential effects that has from one specialty to the next. That both the decline in performance and the longer term capacity implications are concerning is almost without question. But how should a system on its performance knees respond to this increasingly visible reality?

Almost certainly not in the way that it has. In a rather similar vein to the suppression of financial data, we also discovered this week (mid-October 2015) that GPs were to be incentivised not to refer as many patients with suspected cancer into cancer pathways. Quite rightly, clinical professionals were horrified at the glaring conflict of interest in such an important and emotive specialty area, where early detection is the backbone of long-fought improvements in clinical outcomes.

In Summary of Operational Decline

We have now spent more than 12 months, in quarters, missing the 62-day GP cancer referral to treatment target, representing both an operational and a quality effectiveness decline. Additionally, we only occasionally come even close to hitting the A&E 4-hour treatment target and then only because it has been re-set to 95% of patients instead of 98% - itself a form of denial, however welcome the relaxation may have been to Trusts finding themselves the subject of action by regulators.

I have chosen to focus on the generic i.e. system-level figures. However, as you digest those figures you are bound to think about your own Trust. We have to remember that although the generic provides for a very robust sense of 'system health', individual providers may be more or indeed much less healthy that the system.

Therefore, I would encourage you to examine the specific too. For instance, the CCG supervising Worcestershire Acute Hospitals NHS Trust, wrote to its GP population to advise them to cease making elective referrals to the Trust because it was in meltdown. Ironically, that move may exacerbate financial problems for the Trust.

However, it is important to consider the impact of this move on surrounding Trusts. Patients still have rights to care and choices about where to go. University Hospitals Birmingham is just up the road. Previously they have closed their doors, controversially, to out of area referrals. If the next Trust did the same, and the next, we have the very real situation that patients do not have access to care they need. That is a quantum shift in severity of operational delivery issues.

The key conclusion is that it is getting worse. EVERY trend line on operational performance is downwards. Trusts are in operational decline. With this unequivocal reality glaring you in the face, you have to ask yourself just what a further financial stretch target could do. I suspect we will discover that reality over the coming months.

Equally, and perhaps more pertinently to HealthCRASH, these declines are due to an unquestioned increased in demand against a backdrop of poor investment in capacity as providers wrestle with CIP. There is the very real probability that we should have been investing in more capacity in certain areas. My concern is that it takes time to build capacity because of the lag time through training. We may REALLY regret taking a reductionist approach on mass, for multiple years as even if we started capacity building today, it will be years before it shows through. We might not have years before HealthCRASH.

Quality Decline

I have already alluded to the decline in cancer treatment time performance, in which there is little debate as to the impact on people's lives, or deaths, given the correlation between early detection, treatment and outcome. What we don't have is the passage of time for these declines to really start showing in the quality data. However, it would be a gargantuan exercise in denial to have such an unequivocal link established in the medical literature and somehow expect that it miraculously won't show in the outcome data.

Perhaps a more immediate indicator of quality decline, although some will debate the validity and relevance of the findings, is the increase in Trusts being put into Special Measures. To evidence 'decline' as opposed to simply poor performance, it would be useful to have more extensive historical data using the current inspection criteria. In the absence of that, we have an apparent increase in the numbers of hospitals being put into Special Measures, though we also have to appreciate that the ratings are as much about risk of quality and safety failings as they are about actual quality failure.

As a system, we are obviously still smarting from the Mid Staffordshire experience, something we said we must never let happen again. That 'happen' was a catastrophic decline in quality and safety that was precipitated by a cost-reduction set of strategies, resisted by committed clinical staff, who were then bullied to what could only be described as 'submission', leaving the Trust blind to the emergence and continuation of unsafe care. This in turn mediated a financial collapse and Special Measures ultimately resulting in the Trust being put into administration when nobody would or could rescue them.

If that seems like a microcosm of the current NHS story, we'd do well to take heed. After all, we aren't learning the lessons because the exact same story is in its final death throws at Barts Health, with a time and incident course that is near identical. Sadly, despite Barts playing out in full visibility through the media, comparatively few seemed inclined to consider whether they were falling into the same traps and we now have a growing number of equally near-identical scenarios unfolding, not least of which is St George's, another new FT.

If we needed any further evidence, we have to face the uncomfortable truth that Addenbrooke's, centre of the East Anglia Academic Health Science Network and an international centre of excellence, has also been placed into Special Measures. Whereas there has been much debate about whether that was a fair judgement, their own outgoing CEO concluded that 'Needs Improvement' would have been a fairer rating. I think that misses the point. Whereas Special Measures is clearly a disastrous result for a beacon of excellence, a self-determination of 'Needs Improvement' is hardly a quality shift in the right direction for such an esteemed organisation.

At a more anecdotal evidence level, I have been asking the myriad of consultants we work with about their assessment of how under threat quality is and which direction it is going. With very few dissenters, the consistent finding is that we are on a knife edge, only maintained because of the herculean efforts and commitment of an increasingly demoralised and beleaguered staff. That is NOT a quality-stable system, it is a disaster just waiting to happen and although nobody wants to contemplate it, winter this year could just push it over the edge.

As I attempted to quantify the decline in quality and safety, I was actually struck by just how difficult this is as a task. In part that was because of the number of measures that keep changing, making time period based comparison invalid. It would be wrong to say that data measures are changed to prevent trends being apparent but there is no debate as to how difficult it is to draw trend-based conclusions when they are.

An example of this was the examination of complaints, which should act as a good proxy indicator for care quality, given that a stable or improving quality is unlikely to be associated with increasing complaints. Certain data was comparable but recent data contain comparison caveats. However, Figure 8 shows a clear trend towards increasing complaints.

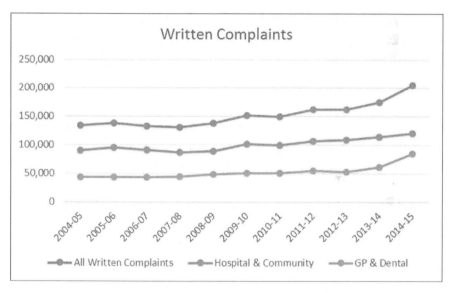

Figure 8. Written Complaints. Source HSCIC.

All of this points to the need for an independent and ongoing assessment of quality, defined in meaningful ways that can provide both time-trend data and comparisons with other healthcare systems. In fact, we do have this: QualityWatch - a joint initiative between the Nuffield Trust and The Health Foundation. It was set up post-Francis in direct response to concerns over quality in an era of huge pressures on NHS finances and delivery capacity i.e. for the exact reasons I am suggesting we need it.

However, QualityWatch can only monitor what is collected and reported and even then only when the data comes out. The challenge they face is the exact same one that I have been facing - the data on quality lags much more than financial data (which comes out <u>ahead</u> of time as a forecast and then immediately on quarter or year-end - providing an immediate comparator too), and that's assuming there is data. So what does QualityWatch have?

The majority of the synopses, tables and reports at the time of writing focused on periods up to around 2011/12 and certainly for international comparisons. I think we all know that we were in a wholly different place in 2011/12 i.e. more stable and less pressured. What we really need to know is what's happening today!

That said, we might just want to reflect that without the additional pressures on our system over the last 3-4 years, we were worse compared to the OECD (western nations really) average in ALL acute care indicators used for comparison (mostly 30-day mortality indicators) and ALL cancer survival and mortality indicators except colorectal cancer. It is also true to say that in the vast majority of these indicators we were also improving. I think an important question that is not answered is whether these long-fought improvements are being genuinely undermined by our current conditions.

Just as I was beginning to consider that I might not be able to draw meaningful conclusions in the area of quality decline, even if anecdotal experience existed, the CQC came to the rescue with its own State of Care Report, released on 15th October 2015. Within their summary, safety was their greatest concern. This was based on rating 13% of hospitals as inadequate for safety, as well as 10% of adult social care services.

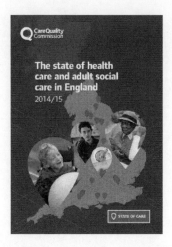

Figure 9. CQC State of Care Report Cover

However, the headline data for inadequate ratings fails to fully capture what has the CQC so concerned. As you can see from Figure 10, a very significant 62 out of 101 hospitals were rated as either inadequate or needs improvement. Given our other evidence of financial and operational decline, along with some evidence of clinical quality & safety decline, the worry is that the 54 'needs improvement' hospitals won't need much pushing to fall into 'inadequate'. The system might struggle if 'everyone' was in Special Measures!

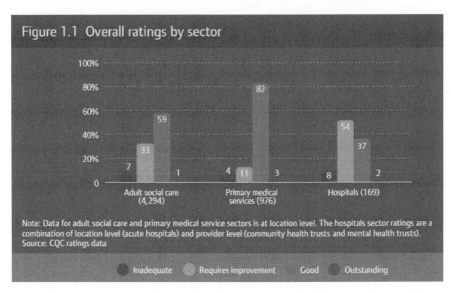

Figure 10. Overall Ratings by Sector. Source & Copyright CQC State of Care Report

To reinforce that worry still further, examining the data on incidents, as shown in Figure 11, we can see a worrying trend towards an increasing rate.

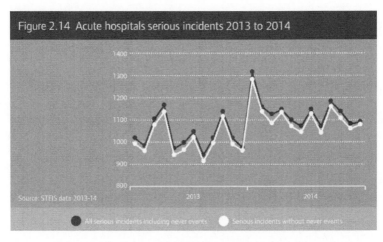

Figure 11. Acute Hospital Serious Incidents. Copyright CQC State of Care Report
Source STEIS data 2013-14

The CQC inspect organisations by care area, by assessing them against a framework of factors. Their findings in these areas and across these factors do nothing to reassure us that quality and safety are not declining. Figure 12 shows quite clearly that 'safe' is the most poorly rated key question.

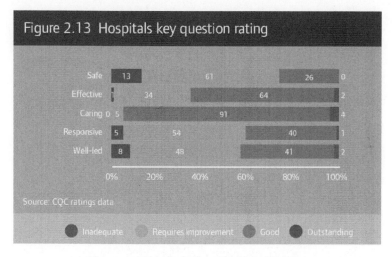

Figure 12. Hospitals Key Question Ratings.
Source & Copyright CQC State of Care Report

When we consider the majority areas of care for a typical hospital, we can see from Figure 13 that medical care is the area of greatest concern, with urgent & emergency care, surgery and outpatients & diagnostic imaging all coming close on the heels and all with over half rated as inadequate or needs improvement.

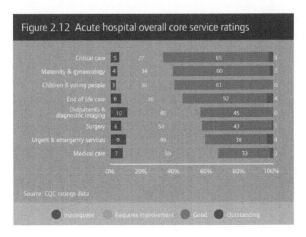

Figure 13. Acute Hospitals Overall Core Service Ratings.
Source & Copyright CQC State of Care Report

Whichever way we look at the evidence, anecdotal or otherwise, we see the signs of system decline in quality and safety. However, given the magnitude of decline in financial and operational performance, I am inclined to say that the quality picture does not show the same catastrophic decline or rate of decline (not that we can assess rate very well). That invites the question why?

Whereas I am sure that most will see the data I have presented as evidence of their worst fears, in truth I wonder if it paints a picture of a profession hanging on for dear life to its most sacrosanct of domains and yet despite that, the cracks are appearing. Whereas the original question - evidence of quality decline - is certainly confirmed, perhaps the more HealthCRASH affirming consideration is in the form of a question.

Taking that picture of precarious safety so clearly demonstrated by the CQC inspections, I wonder what a little bit more financial and operational pressure, coupled to a bit more demand, coupled to increasing complexity will do to our actual performance in this arena?

From my huge amount of time spent 'in the field' with clinical teams, I know that quality and safety are being maintained (in spite of Trust strategies for cost reduction) predominantly through the superhuman efforts of staff. However, I also know just how tired they are. Superhuman effort requires at least adequate energy and will. I can confidently, if anecdotally, report that both energy and will are on the wane and that is something we should be very, very worried about. With that in mind, we need to examine morale.

Decline in Morale

I am perhaps most concerned about morale. And in this we have huge evidence, both anecdotal and factual, as well as of the sort that illustrates the underlying impact too. We are going to run out of staff capacity and it will start (is already starting) with the withdrawal of discretionary effort.

Individuals, not unjustly, are asking themselves whether a loss of their health, well-being and professionalism should be the shattered outcome of ill-thought-through cost-reduction strategies to deal with a problem not of their making. However, this morale-mediated loss of engagement and drive, long predicted by myself and felt through the programmes we run, is symptomatic of a level of decline that has far reaching consequences for our ability to get back out of the poop we now find ourselves in, a matter I will deal with separately. Turning first to the evidence.

A loss of morale, beyond direct measures, is evidenced more by overt behaviour and a few HR metrics such as sickness and absence rates (which have risen in 2 of the last 3 years despite the spectre of job uncertainty and re-grading).

Given that this is designed to be a narrative look at evidence, not a full regurgitation of the actual explicit data (remember, if the narrative made sense, you were going to go check the data in detail to be confident to act), I am going to outline the evidence of decline in morale predominantly from the narrative and anecdotal perspective, based as much on what I am seeing as what the national data from organisations such as NHSIC confirms.

Part of my reason for this as that I am not wholly confident that our primary measure - the National Staff Survey - reliably picks up changes in morale. Whereas the survey is undoubtedly very comprehensive, I think its attention to 'morale' as a distinct issue is very light. That's not so much a criticism as recognition that the survey is not a morale survey. Ironically, having made the case for a more anecdotal discussion, I am going to start with some extremely concerning data.

The Hospital Consultants & Specialists Association, a BMA-like representative body recently (2015) conducted a survey examining stress and its effects across its members. The survey reported results on around 750 established consultants & hospital specialists from a survey request to roughly 3,000 HCSA members, representing a significant sample size, although a survey of its nature will naturally produce a completion bias towards those suffering versus not. That said, overwhelming workload will also have led to many suffering stress not completing the survey too - a balancing factor - and the response rate is already significantly higher than these surveys tend to achieve. The results are stark:

- 68% experiencing unreasonable levels of work stress for half the working week or more

- 71% stating it had taken its toll on their health

- 73% experiencing sleeplessness through thinking about work

- 74% reporting increased workplace stress levels over last year

- 83% confirming that it had impacted on family life

These are not the results of a group with high morale. If morale is high, workload doesn't have the same stressful effects and indeed challenge can be energising. These are not energised people. We have to also consider the group responding.

These are not individuals who entered their profession with any expectations that it wouldn't be incredibly hard work and highly stressful at times. However, despite that expectation at outset, this is how they are reporting their current experiences. We have to understand how bad that is.

More concerning, is what it causes people to do. In the same survey, 81% responded positively to the question of whether they had actively and seriously considered early retirement. Again, we have to put that in context. You have to be of a certain seniority to even view early retirement as a realistic short term option, which probably tells us something about the demographic of the group in this case.

However, early retirement isn't the only behavioural choice for people faced with feeling they must make life-changes to cope with their circumstances. We are seeing these effects in so many arenas and they are all pointing in the same direction - demoralisation of the workforce. These include:

- Rising sickness & absence rates (only held in abeyance by fear of job losses)
- Exponentially increasing applications for Certificates of Current Professional Status, required to work abroad (The Telegraph, September 2015)
- Senior colleagues accepting posts in Middle East, Australia, New Zealand & Canada
- Significant shift to individuals working as locums, rather than substantively
- Increase in working 'to rule' around hours - withdrawal of discretionary effort
- Going part-time but then filling the gap with something more enjoyable or palatable

These trends have been no greater than in an arena we hear so much about - Accident & Emergency Medicine. In a presentation by Clifford Mann, President of the Royal College of Emergency Medicine at the King's Fund in September 2015 and in an article to the Guardian, it emerged that no less than a third (650 doctors) of the medical workforce had resigned in the last three years. Given the enormous challenges to recruitment into A&E and the time taken to produce an experienced senior team member, this is a level of attrition than can only be described as alarming.

We need to remember that the primary question being asked here is whether we are seeing evidence of being in sufficient poop already that this position makes it difficult to get back out in the time we might have available before HealthCRASH. Evidence of this significance is difficult to dispute. That we haven't been tackling this in full crisis mode already is a travesty and indeed more evidence of gargantuan denial in the powers that be. Prediction and forecast of this emerging reality goes back 10 years. We simply haven't acted sufficiently.

If we need any further data confirming the near inevitability of HealthCRASH, it came in a form that should leave the average hospital specialist or senior manager literally grey with concern. Reported by the BMA, the Guardian, Pulse and other media outlets in April 2015, a poll of 15,560 GPs (given we have only 35,000 GPs roughly, we have to consider just how big this is as a sample size) found that 34% intend to stop working by 2020, with many others going part-time or moving abroad.

To add weight to this, we have also seen multiple instances of reported discussions of mass resignations across whole areas in protest to workload, conditions and contractual changes (with most of these concerns being centred on changes that produce more work with less protection).

Given that we are looking for evidence that points towards a significant enough decline in key parameters to predict HealthCRASH, this is evidence enough in its own right but we have to consider where it is going and what its impacts may be. We operate a gate-keeping system in the NHS, as a backbone of ensuring that our universal system is judiciously used. It is reliant on a competent, committed, sufficiently enabled primary care infrastructure.

The Government has pledged 5,000 more GPs in recognition of the importance of primary care to the proper functioning of the NHS. However, it has promised to add them in a single electoral term (yes, I know, you can't produce 5,000 more GPs in an electoral term). This has its own set of implications to the function of gate-keeping, let alone that it doesn't even cover the haemorrhage of GPs we are describing.

If we lose that degree of the most experienced component of primary care, not only are we going to struggle to attract sufficient people in to fill those gaps but we can't do so remotely fast enough, given that rate of attrition. Furthermore, we can't afford to attract them from the limited pool of 'family doctors' in other nations, assuming they even wanted to come to the train wreck that is unfolding in the UK.

The undeniable impact will be a significant increase in demand for secondary care mediated through a decline in gate-keeping robustness. In addition, individuals failing to get access to their normal primary care services are increasingly likely to present themselves to secondary care directly, especially through emergency pathways.

That this is a real and likely effect was eloquently demonstrated by the Health Secretary himself when he circumvented the very system he is purporting to strengthen. In his defence, he said: "I took my own children to an A&E department at the weekend precisely because I did not want to wait until later on to take them to see a GP." And I would say that is the point, poorer access due to insufficient primary care will produce direct presentations.

Whereas My Hunt may choose to say this justifies 7-day GP services, I think it illustrates what happens when everybody has an expectation of something instantaneous that then isn't available instantaneously. Regardless of that difference as a point of opinion, there is the very real problem of how to provide a 7-day GP service when you can't find enough GPs to deliver a 5-day one. There are some answers to this but I will present them in organisational responses to HealthCRASH.

Before moving away from this, I want to close the loop on just how Government plans for primary care have the potential to produce HealthCRASH through the domain of declining morale. The impact is produced via two distinct routes:

- Forcing longer hours and 7-day services into primary care before the human resource is available

- Eroding the gate-keeping quality, resulting in a distinct secondary referral effect

The extension of hours and service entitlement in an insufficiently resourced sector that cannot 'just' fill the gaps is already producing the conditions I have described i.e. the haemorrhage of existing GPs, the suggestion of mass resignation and the massive difficulties in recruiting to a sector that people look at and ask themselves "why would I want to do that to my life?"

To counter those effects, the Government proposes to reduce GP training time to accelerate the availability of more GPs. Quite apart from the very real question of just how we will attract so many more, given the above, this should be frightening to everybody in terms of its implications. The need is not only for more GPs, it is for a competent primary care workforce that judiciously manages the gate into secondary care.

If we backfill the ranks with under-trained, under-experienced GPs, we'll make up the numbers but the effect will be increasing referrals from younger doctors who don't have the confidence and experience to manage risk at a primary care level. The effect of this will be to push up the demand level in secondary care sufficiently to push it 'over the edge'. That edge will be the morale and resilience of the existing workforce. We already know we haven't got sufficient secondary care capacity. We cope 'just' because of the superhuman effort of staff finding ever more innovative ways to shoe-horn more patients through and taking up the excess primarily through discretionary effort.

I don't think it is much of stretch to suggest that if we haven't had HealthCRASH already, this alone would produce it for the secondary care sector. Despite the lack of capacity being reason enough, this added onslaught will be sufficient to cause secondary care doctors to end up with a level of demoralisation and exhaustion that precipitates a massive 'enough's enough' reaction that crashes the system.

All of this is before we consider that, at the time of writing, junior doctors are being balloted for strike action, having just come out onto the streets in London, Nottingham and other locations to protest, and are perhaps feeling more mutinous than many of us have ever seen. Not only is this evidence of their own level of dissatisfaction, it heralds the start of what could be a snowball effect running through staffing groups, even if the genesis of the unrest is different for each.

Despite the absolutely frightening nature of this set of circumstances, ironically I don't think we will have to wait for any of this to exert its full effects to produce that crash. This could almost be viewed as the HealthCRASH back-up plan - if we haven't yet failed financially and operationally, then this will finally do it. And to put it in time context, at the GP-level, that's ALL within a 5 year period - very short in NHS and career terms.

Despite describing this as the final straw backup plan for HealthCRASH, I have spent sufficient time on it because it has very specific implications to question 3 - do we have an ability to get ourselves out of our poop and that is something wholly reliant on staff, their flexibility and their discretionary effort. We will come to that shortly. But first, I want to return to the Government response to its circumstances.

Even though this overt behavioural evidence, just, if not more reliable than a poorly designed national data set, is virtually unequivocal in terms of its severity, rather than listen to it, Mr Hunt's response is primarily to suggest that the BMA are misleading the juniors, that the staff survey suggests that staff experience is improving (or at least stable) and that the Government is actively improving conditions for staff. This is centrally-mediated denial on a positively nuclear scale.

Ultimately, there comes a point when you have to face up to the very real expression of how people are feeling that you see around you, not in the dataset. If the data appears to be different, it is enormously dangerous to ignore the ACTUAL behaviour without first questioning whether the reason for the difference is that your primary measure doesn't adequately assess what you need to be understanding.

We have to be asking ourselves "what am I seeing around me and what does this mean?" and then considering what an appropriate response would be. I believe the meaning is clear. Across many, if not all, clinically-focused staff groups, we are reaching a tipping point in morale, beyond which we will see a staff-mediated collapse in services that are currently primarily held together by the drive and discretionary efforts of those staff.

It is impossible to ignore that the engagement (and indeed continuing employment) of clinical staff is fundamental to being able to provide an adequate health service. I suspect we erroneously believe that they stay partly out of duty and partly out of no choice.

What I am saying is that if we continue with our current cost-squeezing behaviour at the expense of staff, whilst behaving with complete denial around some of the major staffing issues (and consequently not addressing them adequately), we only have to experience a withdrawal of discretionary effort to precipitate HealthCRASH and that's already in evidence.

However, we are seeing the signs of a much greater level of collapse across the workforce and so in terms of our primary question - whether it points towards HealthCRASH - you'd be hard pushed to argue otherwise. The damage is there and we are adding to it, not repairing it, at both a system and organisational level. Both should be very concerned.

In Summary of Question 2

This whole chapter was in response to question 2 of our 4 Horsemen questions - are we seeing evidence of decline in system health sufficient (of sufficient magnitude) to suggest that we are deeply in the poop to a level that suggests climbing out of it will be incredibly difficult. I believe this condition is more than adequately fulfilled. If you'd like a slightly more palatable analogy than climbing out of poop, then it is about the challenges of building sea defences when you are already under water.

I have hardly touched on the evidence of being under water at this moment but it should be clear to all that we are a very long way under water, having been holding our breath for way too long, in a system that is going to demand super-human effort. I would suggest that we have probably exhausted our expiratory reserves and are firmly into residual volume. Not a great place from which to start swimming vigorously.

What's more, I suspect that we have yet to learn the true extent of existing damage. Whereas the figures or evidence of financial decline come out quite early, closely followed by operational evidence, the quality data tends to come out in the wash downstream and the human element is less measurable but no less impactful. On that latter point, I predict we are likely to see a tidal wave overcoming the sea defences (in case you are missing it, the sea defences ARE our committed people).

Our sea defences have been strong but they are built on human resilience, commitment and endurance. This was evidenced by Monitor themselves in their work on last winter, recognising that super-human effort was the primary sea defence. It held... just.

If we remove agency staff flexibilities, add a year of onslaught, increase the demand and complexity a bit more and continue to lambast the sea defences with detrimental pension and tax changes, more crazy more-for-less CIP schemes and other morale-sapping conditions, there is no question that we will see those sea-defences breached.

If we want a further analogy, then the breaking of the levees in New Orleans should remain a stark reminder of just how fast things fall apart when you get a breach of something so instrumental in stability and security. I know we are talking about people, not sea defences, but I challenge you to break that analogy's relevance. On to question three.

Q3. A Question of Capability

Question 3 was about whether we have the capability to produce and implement a solution of sufficient magnitude, sufficiently quickly, so as to avert HealthCRASH. By its very nature, this is a more subjective question than the last one, which was all about evidence.

I am going to suggest from the outset that we just don't know because in truth, to know would mean to have defined the sort of capability we'd need and engage in sufficient research to know whether we had it. We haven't done either, although we have done some.

For instance, the NHS rightly recognised that it needed more senior clinical staff to take on bigger leadership roles as part of a growth in capability to reform. Taking aside the question of how swiftly you can grow the non-clinical leadership and transformation capability and how effective it can be in a system pitched against it, the body of work has produced a fascinating result, if somewhat scary.

The initiative was an NHS Leadership Academy programme to take clinicians with drive and potential, immerse them in development and practical experience, send them to Harvard to augment their knowledge and skills and second them into key positions along their journey. Let's be clear that this is a significant level of investment compared to our typical development programmes. The outcome? Very few of those leaders have taken up significant, influential leadership positions and many have returned to clinical practise.

This is hardly reassuring to our question about whether we have or can grow the capability to lead significant transformation but let's understand why such a significant investment has been so benign in effect (which I take from the personal conversations I have had with a number of the participants). In truth, their journey reinforced to them that the last thing they'd want to do right now is take up a leadership position! That reflects both the immediate prospects and the risk they are seeing or associating with those positions, as well as perhaps something about their view of the senior colleagues they would be joining.

There's an uncomfortable realisation that comes with these findings. The NHS itself recognises it does not have enough leadership capability but it is already in a sufficiently enough damaged state that recruitment and growth of that capability is proving incredibly difficult as those individuals with potential are exposed to the reality. It can't have escaped you that this is further evidence of question 2 - sufficient damage already - but it goes to the heart of whether we can pull ourselves out of where we have gotten to.

Wider Loss of Capability

To reinforce this still further, we have seen a rash of resignations by high profile leaders in recent times, not least of which is Sir Robert Naylor from University College London Hospitals NHS Foundation Trust - one of our historically most stable organisations, at least in recent times. UCLH is anticipating a deficit of around £40 million this financial year (2015), from essentially balance last year.

As we see UCLH staff on our development programmes, they report ever-tightening financial management, vacancy controls, stressed conversations, changing balance of morale and the myriad of other factors that could precipitate the sorts of failures we have seen in Barts Health and others. After 15 years in post, why now, Sir Robert? That's absolutely not a criticism. It's definitely just a question and one which I believe he answered in a post-resignation interview for HSJ.

He graciously cited time for new leadership, whereas many (myself included) might argue that his sort of leadership is exactly what is needed at the current time - stable, steady-handed, with longevity, pragmatic and with a high tendency towards shared or distributed responsibility, rather than the high central control that is part of the problem. Perhaps more poignantly, he discussed a broken tariff system.

This is undoubtedly a major factor in what has produced the deficit in UCLH, an otherwise robust Trust, but I wonder if there is an even more concerning undertone. Sir Robert and other leaders may well be saying that they are concerned as to whether we have the financial, operational and environmental conditions in which organisational leadership, however good, can produce the right results or necessary transformation.

This is a very significant possible conclusion when examining the potential for HealthCRASH because we might be seeing some of our strongest leaders indicating, through their behavioural choices as much as dialogue, that they do not think that 'even they' can produce a successful outcome.

As a result, even great leaders like Sir Robert are very vulnerable at this time. Consequently, perhaps it's time to go, reflecting nothing more than what we are also seeing in consultants, GPs, nurses and other NHS professional groups. Why would we expect CEOs to be different? They are human too.

To be clear, this is not a Sir Robert only issue. We have seen a significant increase in CEO loss to the extent that we now have 14% of posts not filled permanently or about to be vacated (18%, nearly 1 in 5, in Acute Trusts) and 12% of CEOs in post for less than 12 months. That's as much as 25% of the CEO workforce absent or brand new in post - not the perfect position from which to lead radical transformation. Resignations do sometimes come in the vicinity of bad news, such as in Cambridge or Barts Health, but we are seeing the same in otherwise strong Trusts with no clinical concerns, as in UCLH's case. I believe the reasons are clear.

The King's Fund report titled; *Leadership vacancies in the NHS* (December 2014, foreword by Sir Robert Naylor, CEO, UCLH, ironically), described how high executive turnover relates to the risk/reward ratio of these roles. It went on to point out that while the public, politicians and the media all have a legitimate role to play in scrutiny and accountability, when things go wrong, this scrutiny can become intense and be accompanied by blame and disproportionate consequences. That's tough enough in fairly stable times but when times become as tough as they are today, it's a pressure that is proving too much.

Sir Leonard Fenwick CBE, Chief Executive of The Newcastle upon Tyne Hospitals NHS Foundation Trust recently shared his feelings about leading organisations today, citing that the challenges had never been greater and it had never, in all his many years, been tougher to keep things on the straight and narrow. What's more, he described the level of visibility and criticism that leaders experience today as being of a magnitude that made it a very tough job to do in human terms too.

To hold the capability to transform ourselves out of the poop, we have to have the conditions to retain the best leaders with the right capability and drive. We don't. We are currently haemorrhaging them too and unless we change those conditions this will likely grow, not diminish. Even if we change those underlying conditions, we have to see a truly U-turn like reversal of this trend to have the time to do what we need to do.

Insufficient Enablement

To address this question of capability in a more objective manner, we need to be clear about what we might need to achieve what we need to achieve. And we need to achieve a monumental degree of transformation in an eye-wateringly tight timescale, after a long history of failing to do just that.

To help understand what we need that we don't have, I am going to turn to our own ENABLEMENT Model - a conceptual and very practical framework with which to examine any performance or transformation challenge. The premise of the model is that any group of people, whether it's a project group, clinical service or the whole provider sector, needs to be sufficiently 'enabled' to make happen what needs to happen.

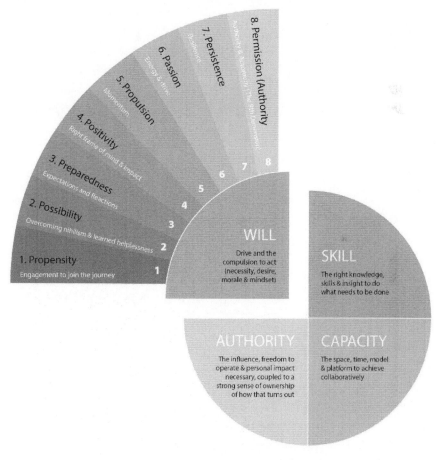

Figure 14. Academyst ENABLEMENT Framework

The ENABLEMENT framework or model illustrates four distinct factors that add up to the capability to do what we need to do. Unfortunately, in each of these we are hugely deficient.

Starting with WILL

Firstly, and starting with the senior leaders themselves, we need the WILL or motivation, compulsion and drive to achieve an enormous agenda that has a high cost of failure for the leaders responsible in leading it. Unfortunately, as I have been laying out, we are losing them left, right and centre and the ones we have are showing a reluctance to do anything radical, even though radical change is exactly what is needed to deal with this magnitude of challenge.

This is not at all surprising, given the high failure rate and 'young' nature of our CEO workforce. Dealing with the significant challenges within an organisation will seem tough enough. However, we are asking for a level of maturity and confidence that allows those CEOs to step back and calmly lead a huge degree of transformation that we haven't fully designed and certainly don't have full agreement over. With the average tenure being just three years, and only 2 years 4 months in the acute sector, we just don't have that maturity.

The already cited King's Fund report also highlighted the very destructive impact of executive loss and use of interims. When it happens, there is a strong tendency for an organisation to lose strategic direction, with interims often not feeling they have the mandate to lead transformation in an organisation they are only with temporarily. Given the current state of play with executive vacancies and the degree of use of interims, we are seeing the perfect conditions for stagnation at a time when we need anything but. If that is scary, let's turn our attention to leadership of clinical services.

Arguably, we have an even greater need for clinical leaders with the right level of WILL or drive, to help lead significant transformation in the way clinical services are delivered. Unfortunately, we have been systematically undermining this through wholly inappropriate responses to difficult times, resulting in a dearth of clinical leaders willing to take on wider roles or engage in significant transformation.

Trusts are finding it increasingly difficult to encourage consultants to take up what many view as a poisoned chalice and where they do have people in post, many are there because it is their turn or nobody else would step up, not because they wanted the position. This is NOT the level of WILL we need to create a monumental effort and solution. What's more, it is going further in the wrong direction.

This finding is fairly unequivocal but I'd like to turn to an aspect that is perhaps more anecdotal. I spend a significant amount of my field-based time with clinical leaders, medical, nursing and managerial. The level of what I will call role babysitting is frightening. This does not mean these leaders are not managing services well but it does point to a huge lack of the WILL necessary to lead significant change in very difficult times.

Again anecdotally, there is a not insignificant body of clinical leaders that are in post to 'protect' their services from the 'evil plans' or inappropriate CIPs of the Trust. Regardless of the appropriateness or not of this position, it points to a level of clinical-managerial divide that is wholly inconsistent with rapid change.

So, we have undermined the very first enabling factor and in reality that alone is enough to undermine what we need, given that this factor is necessary for any of the other factors to even be relevant. Without question we are seeing this at the CEO level but we are also seeing it very firmly at the Service Lead or Clinical Director level and increasingly in other service leadership posts too. Let's turn to SKILL.

The domain of SKILL encompasses knowledge, insight and understanding, not just academic capability and practical skills. At the level of understanding, we are enormously deficient. I am concerned that this alone means that even if we had the right level of WILL, this lack of knowledge, insight and understanding would prevent the right things from happening.

I was concerned enough about this to engage in our own research with 1,500 consultants and then 500 managers, which provided unequivocal proof and realised our worst fears. Presented with 20 multiple choices questions (yes, the answers were in front of them) about how our system was changing, what was driving that, how it worked, how the finances flowed etc, the mean score out of 20 in consultants was 4.8, which rose to the 'thin air' heights of 4.9 when we added in the managers (although financial knowledge went down).

Let's be clear what this is telling us. These are 2,000 senior individuals responsible for leading change, devising solutions and deploying millions of pounds of healthcare resource and their mean level of understanding is little better than random guessing. This is NOT what we need to get ourselves out of deeply complex poop.

It would be wrong to leave SKILL without asking whether we have the necessary knowledge, insight and understanding within our existing senior leaders (those that we have left, that is). This is important because strong, influential, capable senior leaders can compensate for the lack of understanding of those below them, at least to some degree.

Whatever the innate potential, it is clear that it is not being exercised and that could be because it doesn't exist in sufficient quantities. Far from anecdotal, in this we do have some direct evidence. In 2014, the NHS Confederation conducted research with senior leaders and Board members. One question they asked was whether leaders felt that the NHS needed to make substantial changes to maintain current levels of care. Frighteningly, only 51% felt that it did, or nearly half didn't!

This is direct evidence of a woeful dereliction of duty to understand what is actually happening and lead a meaningful response. It also has catastrophic practical implications.

Imagine a Board where, consistent with this evidence, half feel that radical transformation is a necessity and half feel that some more belt-tightening is sufficient. What's the outcome?

Under these conditions, we would absolutely have to have consensus for radical transformation and so in its absence, we continue with the current course of action - belt tightening. The latter causes further damage, including to the WILL of staff below executive level, and the former, necessary for survival, just doesn't gain traction. That alone suggests we do not have what we need in our senior leadership group to produce a meaningful response that actually happens.

What about CAPACITY?

If we are worried already, I think it takes on a whole new level when we consider our third category, that of CAPACITY. Capacity encompasses not only time but also the means to work together on the things that count. Working together on non-clinical issues has become increasingly difficult and as we work with groups they frequently cite the following as confounders:

- No time

- No headspace, even if they have time

- No support for innovation processes

- Little ability to meet in short order

- Difficulty in communicating because of over-reliance on poor email systems

So, if I asked you to 'just' come up with a meaningful solution to deeply complex problems and implement it in a timely fashion before disaster ensues, given the above, how would you rate our chances? We have been running so lean for so long that we have pushed ourselves to a capacity knife-edge and that does not leave us with the capacity we need to lead meaningful transformation swiftly enough.

I see this consistently in the work I do in supporting organisations to move towards clinically-led' (an essential cultural shift to enable us to even push forward solutions that work and happen). Even where Trusts have put in places the structure and authority to allow much greater service autonomy, the leaders of those services, often what we call the triumvirate (lead clinician, matron and manager), have virtually no headspace to do what they need to do.

Although this is clearly a self-fulfilling prophecy, the lack of stability-enhancing leadership and management means that their limited capacity is almost fully eaten up by the ensuing firefighting that comes from a failure to 'get a grip' (in the proper sense of the word). In effect, although we will call them leaders, their non-clinical time is almost entirely operationally focused i.e. managerial in nature. Transformation is something they think about when they have a spare few minutes, which is some when between occasionally and never.

Whichever way you look at capacity, we don't even come close anywhere within our organisations. This is made worse by not having the financial capability or regulator tolerance for slippage in financial or operational performance. In effect, we have got ourselves to balancing on a knife-edge, only held there by relentless here-and-now focus, with a woefully inadequate capacity for anything other than just holding on, in a system that arguably cannot afford to adequately fund change.

Even if the system could afford the financial increase and performance decline necessary for sufficient capacity to engage in rapid transform, it has allowed such an erosion of the capacity-demand balance that we would struggle to even be able to put that capacity back in over a timescale consistent with not crashing. This might potentially mean denying many their constitutional right to elective care within the constitutional timescales, which would require a constitutional change. That alone would prevent that capacity emerging before HealthCRASH was the outcome.

And Finally, AUTHORITY

That leaves us with AUTHORITY - the freedom to operate with a heightened sense of the responsibility or outcome ownership that comes with that freedom. It is true to say that in this domain I am just as worried, although the realist in me says that the lack of what we need in the other ENABLEMENT dimensions renders this a rather moot point. However, having suggested that the move to a distributed leadership environment - the service- or clinically-led organisation - is very much part of the conditions we need to develop, we do need to understand this most important of domains.

Taking aside the complex organisational structures that make it almost impossible to operate with any degree of freedom or authority (an essential component of being able to lead change), we have a regulatory infrastructure and attitude that robs our remaining organisational leaders of what they need to confidently take their own course towards greater stability. I know this assertion will be controversial and the regulators would be first to say that they are positively 'demanding' that leaders act with authority and take charge of transformation. Let's examine what I am getting at.

For instance, the foot-stamping behaviour of the TDA, permitted by NHSE (their boss), makes it abundantly clear to Boards that they are 'not allowed' to permit say 2 years of poorer financial and operational performance as part of a pragmatic approach to creating the capacity to fundamentally redesign. The regulators are saying "we want radical change AND we want operational consistency AND we want financial balance or cost-improvement AND we want absolute safety AND we'll put you in Special Measures or fire you (or both) if you don't do as you are told". We have to be very clear that this does not represent the authority and freedoms necessary to innovate and lead change.

These conditions are certainly no better within organisations. Service leaders find themselves subject to intolerable levels of bureaucratic decision-making, justified on the premise of needing 'grip' in matters such as workforce spend. However, I would assert that this approach to managing internal results is part of the very problem for two distinct reasons that are also at odds with the freedom we need to transform.

Firstly, the elaborate decision-making structures and committees e.g. a workforce panel, create such a single-minded approach to what are genuinely complex decisions that it results in very poor decision-making of a silo nature AND the near-impossibility of fundamentally changing anything.

Secondly, it results in a significant loss of sense of ownership at the service-level, itself leaving Trusts very vulnerable in the safety domain as well as creating a level of clinical disengagement that is completely at odds with rapid transformation, if not any significant transformation.

Rapid adaptability is built on a platform of trust-based decision-making devolved to highly competent individuals with a strong sense of collective direction, purpose and responsibility. I am frequently faced with Trusts reflecting that they cannot just 'trust' their service leaders to make the 'right' decisions and thus they need to control those decisions to maintain 'grip' in their organisation. The lack of insight into what they are articulating is heart-breaking.

Far from not being able to trust individuals who couldn't be more positively intentioned, it is telling them much more about the catastrophic failure by Boards to understand the cultural conditions they need and their role in supporting their establishment. I will often respond with a provocative question; "if you had a group of service leaders who would never knowingly take a decision that didn't fully consider the full balance of critical issues facing a trust (clinical, safety, financial etc) and who had to live with the consequences of that decision on the ground in their service, clinically or financially, why would you ever need a workforce panel and what would ever cause you to think that it would make a better quality of decision?"

The fact that an organisation feels it cannot trust such a positively motivated, intellectually capable and service-owning group of people says so much about the lack of cultural and behavioural understanding in executive teams and the lack of investment in the thinking and understanding necessary in clinical teams, let alone the skills, information and structure. It points to highly complex organisations that might be clinically effective but which are also in a very poor position from a leadership and cultural perspective.

It is clear what needs to happen to change this but we have to recognise our starting point. It isn't that it can't change comparatively swiftly if the right moves are made but we have to consider that we are where we are because this is so poorly understood within organisation. Furthermore, sadly, it is also behaviourally incredibly complex to change, if not impossible, if the wrong steps are taken and we are currently taking those wrong steps with gusto.

I have made it a personal mission to change this understanding but to do so you have to have at least sufficient will in executive teams that they will listen in sufficient depth. Currently they are not, as they run around headless (limbically-driven and blind to their own thinking and behaviour), in organisational death-throws (assuming they haven't already left). My belief is that the majority of organisations will not learn that lesson until it is too late and certainly collectively too late to prevent HealthCRASH. My sadness is that it is so unnecessary and hence my passion to help change it.

Impossible Conditions

I am guessing that you have considered enough already to at least cause you to question whether we have remotely the capacity and capability we need to prevent HealthCRASH. However, there is the need for a brief discussion about whether we have the necessary conditions to support a resolution that prevents the crash. Both capability and conditions are necessary.

By this stage, it becomes increasingly difficult to separate the various component parts or contributing factors in HealthCRASH. All are at play in part, including the magnitude of the influencing factors, the stage we are at already and whether we have the capability we need, as well as the conditions themselves. Considering those conditions e.g. financial conditions, they are themselves complex, given that we create those conditions and they are indeed a function of what is going on that we can't control, interacting with the decisions and actions we have taken to date.

I am not trying to make this discussion overly complex and so to simplify it, we just need to ask ourselves a simply question; "regardless of how they have come to pass and who is responsible, do we have the necessary conditions today to support us climbing back out of the poop we are already in?"

To illustrate that plainly, by opening up one of those conditions, let's look at finance. To be able to create a meaningful solution, arguably we would need some financial headroom. The lack of financial headroom (which very few would argue at this point) is a direct function of our failure to understand what has been happening and take meaningful action. It now becomes another Achilles heel. Whereas financial conditions were only partly causative of the conditions we now find ourselves in, the lack of financial headroom is absolutely part of the difficulty in climbing back out.

I would argue that we need a triumvirate of conditions to genuinely support resolution without HealthCRASH. Furthermore, like all three-legged stools, you only have to remove one leg for the stool to fall over. Those conditions are:

- Financial Headroom

- Time

- Supportive Culture

Additionally, I would further argue we need an intelligent facilitator, which we (not just we) would call a System Architect, who's role would be to focus on the bigger picture and judiciously create and preserve and protect the three conditions above. Arguably, that is the role of Simon Stevens and his NHS England Executive Board but we can't look at that Board without considering that they have created the incredibly unsupportive culture we currently have and are the main perpetrators of no financial headroom.

If we needed further confirmation that a different level of System Architect is needed, it came on the 2nd September 2015 when the Chief Executive himself proudly announced NHSE's flagship policy and approach to the stress and morale disaster facing the NHS - Zumba. This was the very same day that it was reported that DH bailouts had rocketed to £1.2 billion. That £5 million on Zumba, across 1.3 million people (yes, that's about £3.50 per person per annum), is stark illustration that not only does the CEO of the NHS perhaps not understand the issues at play but also that the ideas cupboard is completely bare.

Financial headroom could be provided by the Chancellor, possibly. However, in light of our financial predicament as a country, not just an NHS, his capability is limited, something we are seeing played out in his behaviour too. Furthermore, he would have to overcome the desperately uncomfortable issue of providing yet more money after 'supporting' the NHS through protection and preservation (albeit insufficiently) over and above other sectors of Government spend.

Providing financial headroom now would mean not only savaging other budgets further (or raising taxes, itself not exactly an easy issue for a Tory Government) but providing money in three conceptual tranches where even one of is deeply challenging. I would suggest that what we need is:

- Significant emergency support - that's just for survival

- Restoration of finances back to an even keel, to stop us immediately falling over again

- True headroom from which to lead true transformation

Each of these is an amount almost certainly measured in multiple billions. If the current and emerging data is to be relied on, in truth, underneath all of the rhetoric, we have made essentially zero inroads into the £30 billion shortfall predicted by 2020. To put that figure in context, that's over 75% of the entire defence budget but for the NHS it is JUST the shortfall.

What figure would be necessary to create the right financial conditions for transformation in a timescale that prevented HealthCRASH? Part of the issue is that nobody even agrees. Without pretending to have all that I would need, I would suggest that we briefly examine it in the following categories:

- Emergency get through money

- Restoration of financial security

- Create the right structure & culture money

- Support for transformation fund

First off, we need to relate this to timescales that would allow some stability and prevent HealthCRASH. I am going to suggest that we could, <u>with the right conditions</u>, have undertaken much transformation by around 2020/21 financial year, the magic time point quoted in so many funding discussions, if we appreciate that those conditions are more than money. For instance, we'd need to massively upgrade the culture and degree of understanding, as well as have adequate time to really think through the changes that needed making.

Without a complicated set of financial conditions, many have quoted additional emergency funding in the realm of £2bn per annum. I have no idea whether that's the right figure but we'll use it, given that there is some tacit consensus around it.

In terms of financial security, I am going to use the Nuffield Trust publication from 2012, entitled; *NHS and social care funding: the outlook to 2021/22*. The paper argued that to preserve the long run average we would need to attain approximately an additional £30bn per annum at around 2020/21. That is, of course, the NHS shortfall. In real terms at today's rates, that an additional £90 billion in total over the 6 years, assuming a linear rate of increase.

My third category is more difficult to ascertain and without question, time is the bigger enabler, providing we are vigorously working on it, which would require investment. Assuming we didn't invest the money in some further, slow-moving, more concerned with its appearance than practical benefit arm's length body, I'd estimate around £2bn might be necessary (the purpose here not being to lay out these calculations in microscopic detail).

And finally, there's the headroom to be able to properly support transformation into a form that is sustainable, at least for the foreseeable future, which should be the next 30 years (based on the ONS population projections and peak of the problem). In this we do again have an estimate, helpfully provided by the King's Fund in their July 2015 report titled; *Making change happen: a*

Transformation Fund for the NHS. That report estimated an extra £1.5 to £2.1 billion per annum over that time period, based on tackling the new models of care. At £2 billion per annum, that's a further £12 billion over our 2020/21 timescale.

So, let's consider the reality of what's needed. Assuming we needed emergency support for just one more year, given restoration of financial stability, the UK Government would have to find an additional £106 billion, or just over £17 billion per annum over 6 years. The likelihood of this, given DH assertion that even £2.1 billion (estimated aggregate deficit by Trusts) was unattainable, is so far-fetched that it almost doesn't warrant further discussion.

However, further discussion is required because we are considering HealthCRASH and I am suggesting this is what might be necessary to sensibly transform and have the time to do it, by first creating the right conditions, itself requiring stability. Individuals will look at the figures and think they are la-la land plucked pie-in-the-sky wish list figures. However, they are nothing more than the long run average increase that arguably itself wasn't quite enough, coupled to some emergency support (small), some cultural transformation support (small) and a King's Fund estimated sensible transformation budget.

This demonstrates unequivocally just how far off the mark we really are and hence supports the likelihood of HealthCRASH. If there is a funding constant we face continually around transformation, it's to look at what's really necessary, decide we can't afford it, set something that's a paltry percentage of what we need and then plod on getting ever more stressed that it isn't happening. At some point we might recognise the futility in that and start working in reality. However, having done what we have for so long, whether we could ever do that now prior to HealthCRASH, given current economics, is wildly unlikely.

There's another issue and it is an important one. Let's say for a minute (a brief moment of wishful thinking) that the Chancellor did come up with the cash. That cash would have to be used intelligently and swiftly in the right places and for the right things.

That would require the highest calibre of System Architect, working hand-in-hand, collaboratively with a provider sector that fully understood the circumstances and the transformation imperative. We have none of these and so despite the plight of the NHS, if I were the Chancellor, I'd be very worried I'd be throwing good money after bad.

So, having discussed culture, albeit briefly and finances, fairly extensively, we have to realise that any change would have to be swift and, as a condition, that requires at least adequate human headspace, much deeper understanding and significant development, all of which take time. Perhaps 10 years ago we had time. I would suggest that today we do not, unless we are prepared to put in the sorts of investment I have been discussing. That doesn't just buy development, it buys time for that development and then time for the resulting transformation. Without this, HealthCRASH comes first.

That is illustrated by the current size of the predicament and the rate of change of decline and collapse. To reiterate, the deficit in the first quarter of 20015/16 is greater than the whole year-end deficit in 2014/15, before we get to winter. That rate of decline is astounding. There is no other conclusion.

Sadly, I would suggest that even if we had every other condition, we remain enormously challenged by time. It's not as though the solutions are ideologically, technically, societally easy. There's a very big and difficult conversation to be had about what a 'national' health service could and should be expected to provide in light of the population and economic challenges.

Furthermore, I would argue that we haven't even really begun to discuss a solution, a point I have been making for nearly 10 years now, mostly because of our preoccupation with justifying why we need more funding when the money just isn't there, or hiding the fact that we are uncomfortably where we really are. Time is a prerequisite and it comes with a cost that it appears we just can't afford.

In Summary of our Capability

It is easy to perhaps accuse me of being overly pessimistic but I would argue strongly that to be overly optimistic in the face of what we current have, have not and are experiencing is a form of denial in its own right.

Ironically, I believe we live in an era where there has never been more opportunity but at the same time never more threat. I am optimistic about the future, for those who understand and acknowledge the reality of the present and commit to taking the necessary action to seize a very different future. What I am wholly pessimistic about (and I would describe it as REALISTIC, not pessimistic), is the chances of the NHS escaping without what I describe as HealthCRASH. A positive future requires positive action. That should be a wakeup call.

I have tried to look at our capability to resolve in practical, common-sense, pragmatic ways to provide a framework not only to assess our current capability but also to steer our future direction in strengthening ourselves. I recognise I have hardly scratched the surface but then this was never the remit of this rationale. However, looking at ourselves through these lenses I believe paints a picture of us being near totally devoid of what we need practically, financially and cognitively, to drag ourselves out of crisis in a timescale sufficiently swift to prevent that crisis turning into HealthCRASH.

Of course I don't need to persuade myself and I am not trying to persuade you. I am, though, asking you to reflect on what we have, what we need, the size of the gap and what that is telling you. If that leads you to conclude we are in deep poop, then we had better examine the fourth question - whether someone else will whisk us out of it and clean us off. Unfortunately, as it currently stands, I think we have already partly answered that question.

Q4. Who are the Rescuers?

Part of the difficulty we face is that we aren't just a small group of people, suddenly finding ourselves in a bit of trouble. We are 1.3 million people, in deep, deep trouble and when we look above us, not only are we not filled with confidence, we realise that there isn't much actually 'above' the NHS. It is also of a magnitude that there aren't that many who hold the capability to act as saviours in the traditional sense of the word.

Arguably, unless we sell out to China, we are essentially reliant on one or a combination of three potential rescuers, those being Government, the people and commercial enterprise (I am sure the idealists are already writing their retorts). I am in no way suggesting any course of action. I simply want to look at the possibilities and probabilities. Let's start with the group we believe we elect to save our system - Government.

The Government as Rescuer

I know that I have been providing evidence of the likelihood of Government acting as rescuer as I have addressed other related sections, such as financial position and economics. However, I think it is important to bring some of those arguments back out and in one place. I am going to examine this with our ENABLEMENT Framework, so that we have a good conceptual model with which to consider the possibilities.

For Government to be able to rescue us, they have to want to (WILL), they have to know how to (SKILL), they have to have the time and financial resources to (CAPACITY) and they need to be allowed to (AUTHORITY). It is difficult to know which of these ENABLEMENT factors is present but easy to ascertain which ones are not.

I think we are kidding ourselves if we believe we fully understand the Government's intentions i.e. WILL. Mr Hunt has recently re-iterated that he would like the Tory Party to be the Party of the NHS. However, his actions would either lead us to conclude complete ineptitude or an underlying different viewpoint (or both, of course). What we do know is that the current party is committed to reducing the size of the state in relation to our economic capability, and 'The State' would, of course, include the NHS.

What we can be fairly clear on is that Mr Hunt alone doesn't have the financial capacity at his disposal to rescue us. I would question whether the Chancellor does either without raising taxation and that's before we address whether he would be prepared to. Without the financial capacity and the time it might bring, we can pretty much rule out the Government as rescuer before we even get to AUTHORITY.

I have suggested that the solution may well be an unpalatable but necessary change in funding model for the NHS. That could be a departure from free-at-the-point-of-delivery in favour of a different arrangement such as co-payment, part payment of elective care, insurance etc. It could be restricting scope, which is simply a version of the above too, as whatever isn't provided by the NHS becomes the subject of insurance, private provision etc.

The big question is whether the current Government could (be allowed to, have the AUTHORITY to) carry a change in model in a timescale that prevents HealthCRASH. That would require a population that fully understood the issues and at this point I would strongly suggest they don't, a condition largely perpetuated by recent Governments. Unfortunately, that would also make a sudden Government U-turn on health policy, underpinned by sudden 'honesty' about the true underlying state of the NHS, quite a difficult 'sell' that at best undermines trust.

In the absence of a supportive and permitting population, the most likely outcome of a suggested change is extended debate about what it should be. The last debate on fundamental changes, which stopped well short of a funding model change, took in excess of 10 years to have. That could be shortened by the presence of HealthCRASH but then that proves my original premise - we are heading into HealthCRASH.

I would suggest that the population, from its current low base of understanding, would need to actually feel the loss of healthcare provision when they needed it to simply believe we had that radical a problem, requiring that radical a solution. The deeply disturbing realisation is that this 'loss' of provision is a life-affecting scenario and of course nobody wants that. Consequently, it appears that we need catastrophic conditions to leverage real change and yet nobody wants the conditions to emerge.

It's the equivalent of somebody needing a heart attack to fully 'get' quite how deep the problems are and how urgently change is needed. The problem is that you don't always survive a heart attack and that's definitely true of political parties and especially ones that might need to raise taxes.

To add weight to the conclusion that the Chancellor will not want to raise taxes, we have the growth of support for more left-wing politicians such as Jeremy Corbyn, elected on an anti-austerity mandate. Regardless of anybody's political beliefs or inclinations, this highlights a simply gargantuan lack of understanding of the underlying state of the economy by the population.

That the population might be thinking that we have a <u>strong</u> economy that has been built on austerity leads me to believe that they are also highly unlikely to want to support what is, in effect, more personal austerity i.e. higher taxes. In effect, they are saying we feel austerity personally and we don't accept it. That puts Government between a rock and a hard place when coming to the rescue.

It is also very easy to hold a view that "we oppose austerity" if you are sufficiently ill-informed, or as likely sufficiently misled, as to believe that it is simply a political choice, not an economic reality. However, the reality is very clearly a sufficiently low level of understanding that it would make it nigh on impossible for Government (of any political persuasion) to do what it needs to do.

The reality is that we do not have a strong economy and this invites the conclusion that austerity is simply a function of terrible national economics, not an ideological difference between left and right (although it can be both, of course). I can't possibly address the latter but there is no question that we have the former - very poor underlying economic conditions.

A move from austerity to more heavily support the NHS has to be supportable by something. Support for the Health Service has to come from somewhere. And currently, it looks like the Government, therefore, is not actually in a position to be rescuer financially, even if they need or want to be politically.

Another Government as Rescuer

So, if not this Government, what about another? This is as much a question of time and political change mechanism as it is intention. Our Conservative Government is currently less than 6 months in to a fixed five year term. To consider whether we might see another Government not only take over but do so in time to rescue the NHS, we'd have to consider how a change of Government could possible come to pass within an electoral term that has so long to run and indeed whether that change is at all likely.

Whereas Mr Corbyn would undoubtedly have more open ears to the need to support a national institution with greater funding, we have to consider a.) whether he would have any greater actual capability to provide funds than the current Government and b.) whether he is personally stable enough to carry a Labour Government into power. He is, after all, not without an insignificant number of opponents within his own party.

However, far more impactful is that it would have to take a failure of this Government for Mr Corbyn to even have the chance to lead Labour into power anytime soon.

Despite this, I am inclined to believe that this is possible, despite the Conservative's strong mandate, with the NHS as the precipitating factor. However, again I would have to say that it would take HealthCRASH to precipitate a no-confidence vote of sufficient strength to change Government early in a fixed term and thus the premise of HealthCRASH is proven i.e. this wouldn't prevent it. In the absence of something of that magnitude, I struggle to see the likelihood of a change of Government.

The Population as Rescuer

Arguably, the ability of Government to rescue the NHS is function of the willingness and capability of the population to do so. There is much they could do, from providing taxation income to taking better charge of their own health. At a short term practical level, it could involve turning up for the things they are booked in to, taking the medications prescribed and learning to attend a better selection of places for their less than severe emergency needs (perhaps starting with Mr Hunt himself).

All of this requires a level of understanding that I am not sure they have and someone to lead them that I don't think we have either. It would require a meaningful set of places to go, a public health campaign of huge proportions (given that Public Health England has just had its budget reduced), the willingness and even ability for providers to say 'no' we aren't the right location for you and ideally a robust primary care infrastructure with more than 5 minutes per patient.

Ultimately, whatever healthcare provisions emerge out of HealthCRASH, and I think they will be different to the current funding arrangements, they will need to be supported by a population. If those provisions contain personal implications, such as top up for higher quality tier organisations, or co-payment for elective care, then quality, safety, experience, access time and reputation become even more critical than they are now. This is already a poorly understood area by providers.

Historically, our existing institutions and their myriad of practising professionals have held the belief that the population wants to support them and see them survive, as opposed to seeing commercial organisations come in and take over. However, I would like everybody to consider the likely disconnect between belief and reality, if the immediately preceding experience is one of broken services, increasingly stressed, staffed by ever less caring and compassionate clinical teams and where access time has grown and grown.

Unfortunately, many provider organisations have taken courses of action for cost-saving reasons that undermine staff welfare, safe patient care and a good experience. I have said for some time that undermining the very aspects or factors that you may well rely on for future security is a very swift road to ruin. Unfortunately, not enough have been listening.

This all leads me to believe that the population is not our immediate saviour, except perhaps though Government and yet Government does not have the propensity or capability to be that saviour either. It is important though to remember that population will absolutely be part of a stable future and so we would be ill-advised to continue some of the current strategies that undermine their support.

What about Commercial Rescuers?

So, why not allow larger commercial organisations into healthcare, along with their deeper pockets and huge potential to raise money through the City? Whilst explicitly stating I am ambivalent on this - a neutral commentator - I know that there is a strength of feeling in this that could cause mutiny in its own right. Could we accept rescue from a group that challenges some of the most deep-seated ideological oppositions we have?

I recall the debate between Unison and the then CEO of Circle Health, Ali Parsa, about Circle Health taking over Hinchingbrooke Hospital. It was no surprise that Unison were opposed but Mr Parsa's response was thought-provoking. He asked whether Unison would rather see Hinchingbrooke close than see Circle Health in control. Of course the answer was effectively "neither", a convenient position to adopt when you don't own the problem.

I do believe that the NHS will continue to need commercial organisations and their ability to bring in new sources of money for different forms of delivery model but that they will not be the saviour we need to rescue us prior to HealthCRASH. We have scant resources to adapt our forms of delivery without bringing money from outside Government but there's a real difference between 'participate' and 'rescue', which this section is about.

Ironically, the commercial sector as saviour ceased to be an option when Circle pulled out of their Hinchingbrooke contract. Far from this being the portrayed dodgy dealings of a profit-hungry commercial provider, it was precipitated by the realisation that the NHS was happy to take in commercial millions when it needed it but was not quite as happy with the prospect of providing a return on that investment.

Essentially, the NHS liked the idea of a commercial saviour but never thought through the principles of a workable mandate or contractual arrangements. Every time Circle came close to fulfilling their terms and thus being able to start taking a return, the goal posts were changed. Unfortunately for the NHS, the final time they did this, it pushed Circle outside their terms of reference and they took the option to exit.

Circle have taken an enormous amount of criticism for their exit but I am intrigued why we would expect ANY commercial organisation to be willing to shove in millions of pounds of support but without having any prospect of a return. That's called 'charity' and if that is our desired funding platform for the NHS then it won't involve the commercial sector to any great degree.

As if in confirmation of that very conclusion, and even shortly before Circle exited Hinchingbrooke, another VERY significant healthcare player, Serco, confirmed (in August 2014) that they were going to pull out of the clinical health services market. What had prompted this? Losses of £17.6 million on three of its NHS clinical contracts. Circle were not the first and if the NHS continues to expect charity from their commercial partners, or impossible commercial conditions, they won't be the last. Either way, I just don't see them being saviour whilst we can't give them a good reason to take the risk.

Unfortunately, this leaves us with the final question answered and no other questions to ask that aren't just variations on the theme. If not Government or population or commercial enterprise then who? I have an answer to that but first some important, if uncomfortable, conclusions.

Is HealthCRASH a Likelihood?

I have presented a relatively warts and all synthesis of our current conditions and what they point towards. I have tried to be detached and objective in something that is deeply disturbing and emotionally significant to each of us as individuals, let alone as a group of people with a shared belief in the principles of a National Health Service.

We all rely on the NHS in a multitude of ways, whether it is for care of ourselves and our loved ones, for careers, in business and more. There is very little debate about the outcome we would hope for but it doesn't emerge from hope alone. I prefer to work in reality and am always reminded of the saying "hope for the best, plan for the worst". What worries me is that 'hope for the best' is the predominant strategy in play, not only without much substance but also without much likelihood of being successful. More worrying is how few people have a backup plan!

I recently came across a cartoon of a Board in earnest meeting, with a backdrop of declining metrics behind them and a narrative that ran thus "What if we simply did nothing and something magical just happened?" And that's the predominant behaviour at play that I observe across our system. I would be delighted if something magical happened but I am inclined to suggest that plans and security are perhaps better based on an objective assessment of the circumstances and data.

I presented a conceptual model with which to assess our circumstances. I believe this is important because without it, objectively assessing the state of play and what it means is almost impossible - it just becomes noise and the level of 'noise' is deafening at the moment. If we can't objectively determine, we simply continue to observe and I am absolutely certain that observation alone is not the answer.

The conceptual model was based on four questions. Collectively, these questions addressed whether or not we had the driving conditions to precipitate HealthCRASH, were we seeing the evidence that these conditions were pushing us into significant enough decline that it suggested HealthCRASH, whether we had the wherewithal to get ourselves out of this level of HealthCRASH before a full scale crash and, if not, whether we were likely to be rescued, somehow by someone.

We will all be wanting it to tell us one thing but I think it tells us the other. However much we may want it to be different, I believe that an objective look at the data and circumstances around us pretty much demonstrates that HealthCRASH is inevitable. If that's the case, we had better start turning our attention to the bigger question of what should we do?

Should we try to prevent HealthCRASH and if so, how (and is that even possible, given this diagnosis)?

If it is going to happen and we can't prevent it, what, then, should we be doing? Should it be a personally-protective response or a greater-good response? What should we do if those are mutually exclusive? I am guessing that we are entering very uncomfortable territory for many of us.

As I made perfectly clear at the start, this exploration of the likelihood of HealthCRASH was predominantly just that and not specifically about solutions or distinct courses of action. However, I do believe that to leave you with the strongest of senses that HealthCRASH is a 'when' rather than an 'if' and to then not give you a sense of hope and possibility, I would leave you with a sense of 'hopelessness' and that is wholly inconsistent with the statement I made about there being never more opportunity.

However, I want to deal with a VERY difficult issue and if we aren't willing to address it head on, I can probably direct you to stop reading right now. Why? Because frankly, I'd be wasting my words if this wasn't a resolved issue. What's more, I don't care whether you are a consultant, junior, nurse, manager, NED, executive board member, allied professional, cleaner, commissioner or in the heart of NHS England - the issue is the same for every single one of you. What is it?

I believe there is absolutely no possibility of a largely positive outcome for individuals, GP practices, clinical services, Trusts and NHSE without accepting that we need to DO something and that it must be intelligent and DIFFERENT to what has got us to this point in the first place.

With that in mind, I am always reminded of a quote often attributed to Einstein in one form or another but which may in fact have a different origin. That aside, the quote is a thought-provoking one and one that we should all reflect on. It is: *"The significant problems we have cannot be solved at the same level of thinking with which we created them."* Given our propensity for denial and justification, it is one of the reasons for me concluding that the existing leadership i.e. Government, DH & NHSE are unlikely to come up with a miraculous plan to prevent HealthCRASH.

I want to be clear here. When I am talking about a positive outcome, I am NOT suddenly concluding that we will prevent HealthCRASH. A positive outcome is coming through the crash relatively unscathed personally (personally as an individual, service or Trust), with all the faculties needed for a successful future intact, ready to seize a future which could be radically different to the past, built on different principles and probably a different funding model, at least partly.

Could we Still Prevent HealthCRASH?

In some respects I have already laid out what might need to happen for HealthCRASH to be prevented but for ease of understanding, let's bring that back out in the open in one place. Let's be clear, to prevent it we are going to need a level of 'extreme' that we are unlikely to get until HealthCRASH proves that we need it i.e. until crisis becomes a disaster, until the reality is unignorable. However, let's look at what that might entail.

I want to be honest. I am not qualified to claim that what I will describe is the right or only way. I don't believe that anyone is sufficiently qualified as such to act at the precipice between crisis and disaster because the very nature of what you face, at a system level or organisational one, is extreme and unfolding so quickly that planning is very difficult. There is huge uncertainty. Think, Rudolph Giuliani, waking up one morning with planes parked in towers. He gained enormous respect for his leadership but he'd be the first to admit he wasn't qualified.

Additionally, there is a level of detail or granularity that would have to go into an emergency solution that I do not want to and cannot convey easily here. It doesn't mean that what is about to come is simplistic, purely that detail is not the purpose of this book in this particular subject. What's more, I think that those in power are so unlikely to adopt what they might need to do that it is a waste of words and I am better devoting more detail to guidance in coping and emerging from HealthCRASH than preventing it.

That's not pessimistic, it's realistic and why I have concluded that HealthCRASH is virtually inevitable. If I felt there was a likelihood of a radical change in behaviour at the top, I'd be pushing for it. However, I just see no evidence of it and in fact lots of evidence to the contrary.

Introducing Leadership Potency

So, with that in mind, I am going to turn to another of our leadership models, designed for just such circumstances. It's called the LEADERSHIP POTENCY Framework (LPF) and it is at times like this that we need a potent leadership response.

Leadership Potency is based around the question of what a good leader is really there to do. That is never more important than in a crisis but we have to acknowledge that a good leader is there to prevent difficult circumstances or problems becoming a crisis in the first place. In that, the upper echelons of our system have not been successful at all.

At this point, it would be useful for you to have a full-sized copy of the model, given that you are probably reading this on a Kindle. You can access this freely at:

http://academyst.co.uk/leadership-potency-model

Go on, do it. You'll find it much easier to understand and the schematics will be much clearer. It also has some reflective exercises in it to assist you with your own personal development of Leadership Potency.

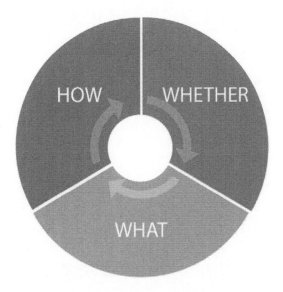

Figure 15. Simplified Leadership Potency Framework

The LPF is based around 3 core principles, illustrated by Figure 15, those being:

Determining WHETHER something needs changing, solving or addressing - to stimulate steady-handed action in a timely enough fashion in things that have consequences if ignored. What goes into WHETHER is captured in Figure 16.

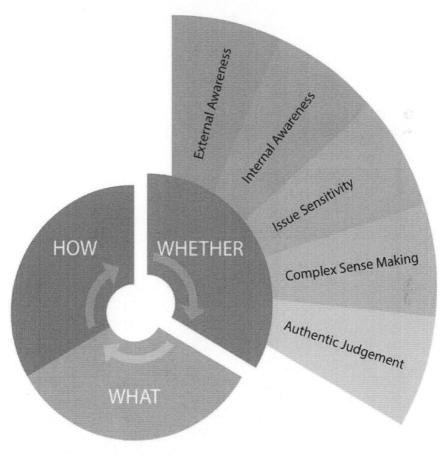

Figure 16. LPF - WHETHER Break Out

The process of determining WHAT actually needs doing - to establish an appropriate and sensible solution to the issue at hand that is actionable and of the right magnitude. What produces the right WHAT is captured in Figure 17.

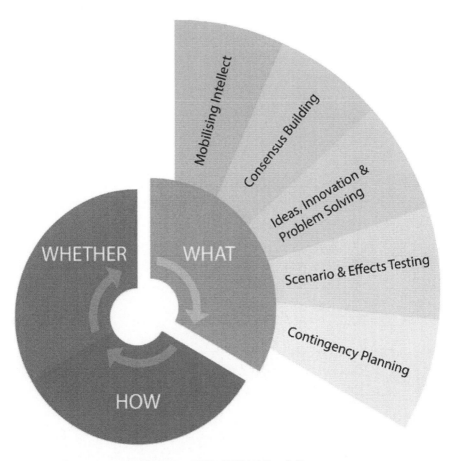

Figure 17. LPF - WHAT Break Out

Leading an approach to the HOW that actually creates the right momentum and action - to ensure that the group, service or organisation acts & adapts proactively with both drive and alignment. That HOW, illustrated by Figure 18, is a reflection of our ENABLEMENT model, already discussed.

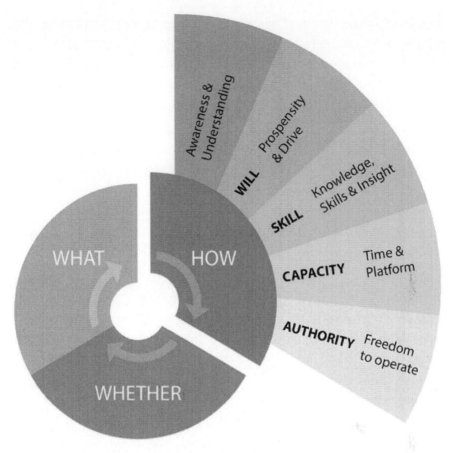

Figure 18. LPF - HOW Break Out

The fact that we are discussing the probable inevitability of HealthCRASH is indication at just how much we have failed both WHETHER and WHAT. An early WHETHER response gives you time to do something well-planned and steady-handed. We are well beyond that now, which is why I have said that we probably need an extreme set of actions to actually prevent HealthCRASH.

Whereas it will feel that my 'accusation' is firmly aimed at system and Governmental leaders, it is worth noting that we have a failure in WHETHER potency at all levels - Government, System, Commissioner, Provider (primary, secondary and tertiary) and individual. How many Trusts are continuing to perpetuate the death-cycle that is more CIP in a bone dry stone? What, as an individual, have you actually done that is different? I am sure that this is an uncomfortable realisation, assuming the denial and defensive reasoning doesn't cut in to save you.

If we need any degree of proof in that, it came from the previously discussed HCSA well-being survey that showed just how high a proportion of individuals were suffering a multitude of very real problems from home and marital difficulties to potentially life-threatening stress-related ailments. To be slightly kinder than perhaps I have been, it is extremely difficult to get WHETHER right, especially timing, but nigh on impossible if you don't systematically look at the evidence with a good conceptual framework.

Arguably that's the core purpose of the book - to provide you with sufficient evidence with which to draw a meaningful conclusion, along with the conceptual framework through which you can examine it. Anyone that reacts poorly to the need for a 'model' is denying just how important a model is for making sense of things. We do need the right models though!

Our lateness on WHETHER makes our choice of our WHAT actions and solutions all the more important. A good analogy for this is found in the dissections of the Ebola crisis, another profound example of a failure to determine early enough that something very different needed doing. The double calamity within Ebola was that when it was firmly established i.e. unignorable, that we needed a radical response, the response designed was more cautious than radical. That left Ebola in charge for way too long, with devastating consequences.

When considering WHAT, we need to consider three dimensions; the actual 'what' obviously, as well as the magnitude of response and how fast we need to engage in it to prevent further, unrecoverable destruction. In the Ebola crisis, eventually the response was of the right magnitude and yet all who were involved will admit it was late and they got away very lightly compared to what was about to unfold when the World got involved. We need to think in a similar manner. What will happen if we don't 'all' engage in a more radical solution, fast?

Finally, I wish to say very little about HOW, other than to state very strongly that the organisations that prevail will be ones that do so with and through their staff, not in spite of them. That should be a massive wake-up call for many a provider, with so many hell bent on more-for-less strategies with staff changes as the backbone, and if you are sat there thinking you have no choice then I would urge you to look in the mirror at just how much you really have the necessary leadership capability, or not.

Preventing HealthCRASH

So, to reiterate, I think there is a small window in which we could engage in a sufficiently radical enough course of action that HealthCRASH could be prevented. It would have to be built on the back of an immediate acceptance and indeed consensus of the massive likelihood of HealthCRASH, or we just won't end up with sufficient drive.

In terms of the size of that small window, I would have to express deep concern over the impact of this winter, just around the corner. We survived last winter, according to Monitor (and I agree), on Herculean effort and a high level of agency staff, along with cancelling much of the elective caseload. Unfortunately the latter will help precipitate the financially-mediated parts of HealthCRASH, even if it helps get through the immediate crisis.

This year, we are entering what is supposed to be the most severe winter for 50 years, with freak ocean cooling in the Atlantic threatening to trigger a nationwide whiteout. Emergency services have been warned to prepare for what is likely to be a repeat of the 1962/63 winter which saw rivers and lakes freeze over across Britain and has already produced shock warnings and fears that Britain could face fuel and food shortages as roads and transport networks grind to a halt. This is not the time to be 'seeing how well the NHS copes' with a cap on agency staff.

If (and the Met Office seems to think 'when') this happens, we will be facing a significant increase in demand, especially around frail, elderly people (who produce the greatest demands on actual care input) on the back of worse finances and lower staff morale (and thus a lower likelihood of the same Herculean effort). Consequently, I think that some of the changes we need to make have a timespan of weeks, not months or years, uncomfortable though that is.

So, if we agreed that we were about to enter HealthCRASH and that its consequences would be grave and that this Winter could well be the straw that breaks the camel's back, then what would we need to do. It would require a two-stage response - immediately and very soon on the heels of immediately.

The immediate response would have to be about winter readiness and survival. That might entail a forgoing of the agency caps to support services that need to mobilise greater numbers of staff than they currently have to cope with emergency load. That could mean utilising experienced and capable staff from across all services and back-filling their essential but less complex care with perhaps agency staff who can cope with it.

We will need capacity, a tough issue when many a secondary care organisation has been reducing it. What could we re-open? Where else could we get it from? I have two thoughts on that latter question, both involving traditionally non-secondary care locations.

The first is to be prepared to support a much heightened level of care in care homes of one form or another. We know they have a 40-50% higher admission rate through emergency pathways than an age-matched non-care home population and although that will partly be driven by a difference in average healthcare status too, the reality is what it is and we can start to address it at source.

The second is to investigate and have on hand a range of hotels (quieter in the winter anyway) that we could call on for step-down care and to support recovery in functionally stable patients. UCLH utilised the Grafton Hotel on Tottenham Court Road for just such a purpose for a number of years.

Both of the above suggestions require mobilising healthcare teams in different ways - the home team, the care home team and the team that supports in ad hoc locations. That's not easy on insufficient nurses already but then it doesn't all have to be nurses!

Capacity would again be gained by cancellation of elective case load and organisations should be very much thinking about 'which' case load to preserve and which to cancel. It's a poor response to cancel across the board, evenly, without considering which caseload has the least or greatest financial impact.

I would also urge organisations to work out what initiatives and processes need to be let go of in the short term. A core failing in a crisis is trying to maintain everything and thus making it very difficult to do what's truly necessary. That would require a massive upgrade in thinking and crisis readiness to ensure that the functional area leaders were empowered with freedom to operate but understood what they were allowed to do or not and how to think about the freedoms to operate with overall stewardship.

Finally, there is a role that Government needs to play. Currently we have regulators literally screaming at providers not to spend a penny more and indeed cut still further, as well as demanding attention and data as though they are the most important part of staying on the straight and narrow. If that position is maintained, it is wholly inconsistent with preventing a crash this winter.

Consequently, not only do the hounds need calling off but the system needs to immediately have a similar leadership conversation with all Boards about what they can and can't do that allows them to adequately deal with the crisis. They need freedom to operate. They handle crises of a winter nature well and have proved that. This year they need more freedom to move and that includes financial freedom without having to worry about personal job security at the end of it.

Government must find sufficient money for a pause whilst we get through this winter. That's more than just winter pressure money, it's money sufficient to take the issue of money off the table, so that we can concentrate on the more important issue of getting through without a large-scale disaster. That will be uncomfortably affordable but it will be painful and it needs bearing.

So, if that gets us through to spring, what do we then need to do?

I believe we then need 5 years to effect a complex set of changes that are in effect not yet designed, certainly not fully. However, those changes need to be enacted in a system that is able to change sensibly, or any design, good, bad or mediocre, will fail at implementation phase. That requires an intelligent system architect and we had better think carefully who that should be. We do not have that architect or change capacity at present. It needs building urgently.

At this point, I want to raise a danger. The minute that Government digs deep, assuming they even can, and provides us with a financial window, we run the risk of breathing a sigh of relief and sitting back somewhat. It's akin to being in a horrendous storm in which we get a lull. There's a reason we talk about 'lulled' into a false sense of security. The greatest danger of the window, is that it risks inertia and inaction creeping back in. We ALL need to appreciate that this is a period where it is incumbent on us all (where we are morally obliged) to fully understand what is needed, understanding our individual parts and get stuck into it with gusto.

To be clear, if we spend 5 years discussing the ideology before we even start to do anything meaningful, we will have missed that window. It will probably require some uncomfortable changes to the funding model, from higher taxes to co-payments or the like. There will need to be an urgent and honest conversation with the population. The current Government could well be a casualty but the need is more pressing than the sensibilities.

I have also previously described what I think it would take financially - £106 billion over a 6-year period. The enormity of this cannot be underestimated. There's a huge danger to trying to undertake this level of change without sufficient financial headroom with which to do it. It's a lesson we are already learning the hard way and is partly causative in our current conditions. If we try to do it 'on the cheap' it just might not happen at all. And that would be the most expensive thing of all to let happen.

There's a chronology to this that we mustn't ignore. It goes to the heart of anything being actionable. For large scale change to happen, it needs to be ENABLED i.e. the people who will participate in it, from top to bottom, need to have the WILL - the motivation, compulsion and drive, the SKILL - knowledge, skills, insight and understanding, the CAPACITY - time, money & facilitated process, and AUTHORITY. Enablement is not a linear process but it does all start with WILL and this comes from a common understanding.

Consequently, the route to preventing HealthCRASH probably looks like this:

1. First, focus on surviving winter, something on which we have reasonable consensus on how to do, despite the regulator mixed messages.

2. Ensure that everybody (including the population too) agrees on the need for radical transformative action and the consequences of not engaging in it i.e. consensus on the magnitude and urgency of what we are facing (hopefully this book with help)

3. Engage in transformation to the service-led organisation (to provide the cultural conditions for rapid adaptability and the basis with which to lead change when you don't have explicit authority), with adequate support and a clear, agreed picture of what that is (much more later)

4. Build a level of transformational change capability, based on a true understanding of the behavioural complexity, not just the technical process (concurrent with 3)

5. Agree a series of national options, or combinations thereof, and undertake a process of consensus building over how well these address the true nature of the problem in all its complexity, allowing a singular choice of components to be decided upon (started concurrently with 3 and 4)

6. Systematically change, rapidly, with full engagement of everybody and probably zero tolerance for those that won't assuming the other 5 steps have been engaged in to the full spirit of their intention.

Even with this conceptually better approach, there are still huge difficulties. For instance, we have a host of existing contractual arrangements that make it difficult to back-track out of what we have, let alone move forward. PFI is a classic example. The overall level of understanding is wilfully low, including at the highest levels. We have official bodies that would feel threatened by some of the changes i.e. would respond limbically. And, not least of which, we have a population largely in the dark of the healthcare tsunami they are going to be hit with.

We have organisations that are exerting tighter and tighter control, in the interests of maintaining 'grip', where we need a devolution and distribution of decision-making towards the clinically-led or service-led organisation. However, we also need services with the capability to step up, act with genuine stewardship and know what to do. That's a behavioural tangle of immense proportions.

We have to overcome the issue that Government, NHSE and Boards believe they are granted AUTHORITY by mandate and yet fail to recognise that if they cannot produce what they intend by 'instructing' people in what to do, this type of authority is worthless, if not dangerous. Unless we are going to disassemble the morale and ethical backbone of a safe system - medical and nursing advocacy for the patient - we have to shift from authority to consensus as our way of getting things done.

That this is all difficult to grasp is an understatement. The likelihood of Government understanding their errors, being willing to make a policy U-turn and being prepared to extract cash from other sources regardless of the onslaught of criticism that brings is slight. Without the window that they can provide, I am inclined to think that HealthCRASH is inevitable and I am deeply concerned that this winter will be a deciding factor.

A Moment of Reflection

I fully realise that the conclusion that we are almost inevitably likely to be entering HealthCRASH is depressing and we'd love it to be different. However, we need to understand that HealthCRASH isn't necessarily a crisis for everybody but it does have huge consequences for those not appreciating it and acting accordingly. More worrying is that it has the potential to affect many lives, from a career perspective AND from a health perspective. I think we all have responsibilities in that, to mitigate the adverse effects.

Finally, before we switch from conclusions to guidance, I know that some will even be suggesting that the very presence of this book could precipitate HealthCRASH by the behaviours it incites. I would hope that the majority see that for what it is - a form of denial. I have not created the conditions and evidence I have described. Those conditions do not change because I have written them down in one place. They are what they are and it is those conditions that determine the likelihood of HealthCRASH, not the description of those conditions.

My concern has always been that we are walking headlong and blindly into HealthCRASH and that allows the powers that be to quietly absolve themselves of responsibility, blaming circumstances instead of their lack of willingness to openly face and act to mitigate. That can't happen if the true nature and complexity of the problem is 'out there' for all to see.

Hopefully, if this book achieves anything, it will be to ensure that 'not acting (differently)' ceases to be an acceptable option for anybody. I remember a meeting on stroke reforms where somebody asked the very provocative question along the lines of "given that we know what the problem is and how many people are dying unnecessarily, at what point do we become responsible for NOT making this happen?" I think a similar question is applicable to HealthCRASH.

That uncomfortably said, it should leave us all with a very strong sense that doing nothing is now off the table. We all have responsibilities. Those responsibilities are to our organisations, the system and to the very patients everybody serves when they participate in that system. However, they are also to ourselves (our health and security) and to our families.

There's a very positive outcome that could emerge from aligning those interests. Presently they are not in alignment and that is adding to the problem. When Government devolves budget to a council, we have to ask whether that's alignment or political protection. When a Trust squeezes more blood out of its human resource stone, knowing it is already at breaking point, it is not alignment, it is saving one at the expense of the other.

At an individual level this is a difficult dilemma. You are employed by the very people who engage in the above. However, I have one question - just how much are you willing to forego the integrity of patient care, your own health and your family security IF (and the IF is important), your organisation and the system do not do the right things?

Consequently, I am going to address guidance from the perspective that HealthCRASH doesn't need to affect everybody in the same way. Those that learn to do the right things for the future and/ or what's necessary for security in the near-term will likely have a safer passage through HealthCRASH than those that don't.

And with that, we should get on with guidance, remembering that a granular solution was never the premise of this book. I am saying that I do not want us to lose the core purpose - a determination of whether HealthCRASH was a possibility or maybe a probability.

An Important Personal Moment

With that in mind, I am now going to ask you to stop for a moment. Don't read any more at this point (maybe to the end of this suggestion)! I'd like you to reflect on what I have described with no requirement beyond reaching a conclusion on whether you believe that HealthCRASH is a possibility or probability and if so, when it is likely.

Think about the four questions - whether the challenges we face are deep enough to precipitate HealthCRASH, whether the damage we have already suffered is severe enough, whether we are sufficiently devoid of what we really need to get ourselves out of the poop and whether, if we can't get out, someone is likely to just rescue us. Thinking about all of this:

What's it telling you?

How do you feel about it and why?

How certain are you?

What would you need to be more so?

How acceptable is 'no action' to you?

What does it mean to you, personally?

These are important reflections. We are about to step into guidance. It shouldn't matter who you are and where you sit in the overall hierarchy, there will be things you need to do and things you should do. However, before any action there should be a decision that action is necessary.

I will leave you reflecting though that a NO ACTION is also a decision. It's a decision with the same culpability as a decision to do something. However, in this case, it's a decision to accept the consequences that emerge from doing nothing, when something is warranted.

When you have reflected on the above, and come to a decision, I'd love to know what it is, either way. Please take a moment to visit HealthCRASH.co.uk and let me know. I absolutely promise to hold that view confidentially. You can do this at:

http://healthcrash.co.uk/my-view-on-healthcrash-likelihood/

As a result, you'll be able to see collectively what people are saying and I'll keep you informed as things unfold.

Time to reflect...

Guidance on Facing HealthCRASH

Welcome back. I am guessing that if you are still reading then you decided there was some substance and thus you needed to start considering how to act and what to do. So, let's get on with just that.

From the outset, I want to make two things clear, both of which are consistent with sensibly approaching a crisis that could turn into a disaster.

The first is that this guidance is firmly rooted in the assumption that we will be entering HealthCRASH as a system i.e. prevention of HealthCRASH from a system perspective is not the focus. I have, of course, already dealt with that in the previous section.

The second is that in a crisis, matters unfold rapidly and a sensible course of action all the way through to the other side isn't usually obvious at outset (otherwise everybody would be taking it). Consequently, some of the guidance is about how to behave and react, not necessarily explicitly what you should do. That doesn't mean I don't know. It means that ANYBODY saying they do know is falling into the first crisis trap - of believing they have all the answers. They don't, and that makes your ongoing behaviour all the more important.

The guidance I have to give depends on who you are and from what perspective you are reading. It is in outline only - assuming that WHETHER is now a done deal, my guidance is going to focus on WHAT and not so much HOW (or we'll be in the thick of HealthCRASH before I've even released the book).

There are things I think individuals need to do and there are things that I think leaders need to do, accepting that they are one and the same at the end of the day. My guidance falls into three categories and they are all centred on the distinct possibility that what starts out as a gargantuan crisis i.e. HealthCRASH, turns into an unmitigated disaster if we take the wrong steps. What constitutes disaster is likely to be different from one person or service to the next.

We should all be mindful of one very specific thought. Whatever kind of disaster emerges for individuals, services and Trusts, it is tiny compared to how it may affect patients at their times of greatest need. It should be an imperative for each of us to never forget that ourselves and never let it be forgotten by those more distant from individual patients.

I also want to start with a small word of warning. The likelihood is that most will not realise what they need to do until it is too late. I am sure you are aware of the saying about leading a horse to water. Too many will continue reading from a perspective of "that's interesting" without really getting that it is YOU who needs to do something.

Give Fish or Teach Fishing?

There is a short saying that I think is quite pertinent to responding in a crisis and it goes; *Give a man a fish, feed him for a day. Teach a man to fish, feed him for a lifetime.* This goes to the heart of my 10+ year quest to foster understanding in these issues and the sort of changes that make for a stable future i.e. an ability to fish. This is in stark contrast to the help we tend to draw on i.e. that of a typical set of management consultants, who feed themselves by providing enough fish for you to feel satiated but not the ability to fish, which might make them redundant.

I think we have to realise that we are way past the capability to keep wheeling in a big consultancy that looks at the wrong part of the problem in the wrong way and then charges you £4 million for the privilege with no true accountability as to whether it makes a long term difference. If you are to survive and indeed thrive out of HealthCRASH it will come from urgently learning how to take charge of your own destiny rather than relying on others.

I am pretty sure that is actually a welcome message to those that find themselves on the end of an ill-conceived solution to the wrong problem, a problem they understood better themselves anyway.

The good news is that we have a degree of intellectual capability at our disposal WITHIN our Trusts that is the envy of any industry and we need to start there by ENABLING it. To do so, we have to also learn how to stop turning it off. We also have to understand that accessing it relates to a combination of structure and behaviour that collectively add up to clinically-led. If you really took the trouble to understand the pieces, you'd also understand that this isn't just a view, it's a ground-zero necessity.

It also requires nurturing in a very specific manner, with a very specific set of operational and governance issues resolving too. There's a combination of structure, process, behaviour, interaction, focus and skills that add up to a workable platform within a provider. It's not a menu, at least not an *à la carte* one. Perhaps I would be better describing it as a fixed menu - leave out a course and you are disappointed by the results.

I am raising this for two reasons, one from a provider organisation perspective and one from an individual one.

As an organisation, making this transition, in deeply troubled times or otherwise, it is partly a survival necessity and partly your route to a secure, prosperous future. There comes a point where you need to recognise that running around ever more headless but without the transformation conditions being present on the ground, only makes matters worse, by further eroding motivation, drive, morale and support.

I am saying here that you NEED to change this and in short order so that you are leading crisis readiness and longer term transformation with and through staff, not in spite of them. Mentally and physically killing them, causing them to withdraw their discretionary effort, causing them to leave and at 'best' resulting in them just working to rule is part of the problem not the solution.

Let's be clear here, I am giving you the baseline conditions to learn how to fish as an organisation. Why? Because system and regulators are not going to bail you out with enough fish and typical management consultants are predominantly going to want an unfair share of the fish for the level of benefit returned. You need to learn how to fish and in a way that genuinely catches enough fish.

At an individual level, I think there are two very important considerations.

Firstly, do you work for an organisation that wants to learn to be different or just keeps perpetuating the same? When things don't work or they encounter resistance, do they push harder, or listen harder? Are they largely reactive, or predominantly proactive and steady-handed? Do they seek to influence their conditions or just respond to what those conditions produce?

I raise this because it is vital to determine this to know what to do. Also, it is worth considering whether they know any better. If that's a concern, expose them to better understanding and see if they change. If they do not, you have your answer.

The question I would ask you (have asked you already) is; to what degree are you willing to put your health, well-being and family at risk for an organisation that isn't willing to show the same commitment to its family? This is a fundamental question and one where the answer determines just how hard you'll work to preserve that organisation, probably requiring you to dig deeper still, versus how important it might be to preserve yourself. You cannot carry the Trust's ongoing failure to learn on your shoulders through something as severe as HealthCRASH.

Secondly, regardless of the outcome of that vital question, you cannot let go of your own security and well-being. That does not constitute surviving HealthCRASH. Whatever we end up with on the other side, it will require high functioning, enthusiastic and committed professionals, whether they be medical, surgical, diagnostic, allied, nursing, managerial or whatever. It's a double disaster if we get to the other side and everybody we now need is burnt out or in Australia.

In summary, if you run an organisation, you are going to need your people on your side. It is very much time to learn how to succeed in that. If you are an individual, support organisations who choose to learn how to take that road and regardless of the organisational road taken, always look after yourself at least sufficiently that you too can emerge, regardless of whether they do. You are not serving your patients or any patients to end up unable or unwilling to care for them.

Three Types of Mitigation

Let's start with three categories of guidance and understand them in relation to HealthCRASH. Then we can explore them in greater detail. They are:

- Disaster Aversion

- Disaster Preparation

- Disaster Recovery

An early word of caution. It is possible to look at these and see a set of if-then scenarios e.g. IF disaster aversion fails, THEN we need to focus on disaster preparation. That's the equivalent of a boat in a storm trying to steer a course to safety but not battening down the hatches at the same time.

This advice is firmly AND, not EITHER/OR and if you feel you can't afford the time, headspace or money now, just consider what that may feel like if you don't engage meaningfully in these things. Even disaster recovery starts now because it is the strongest form of denial to believe that HealthCRASH is probable but it won't affect or touch you. You need to be making sure you have what you need to grow out of the ill-effects in a strong and positive manner.

In disaster aversion, we will look at the sort of things that we might need to engage in or do to ensure that even though HealthCRASH will happen, its effects are not felt to the same degree, if at all, by those organisations that are successful at this.

The ultimate form of system disaster aversion is avoidance of HealthCRASH, a topic I have dealt with at some length and which I feel is not what we should be pinning hope on. Consequently, this is focused on individuals, services and organisations, not the system.

Disaster preparation is about readying ourselves, our services and our organisations, under the assumption that we probably won't escape the storm. This is the equivalent in ship terms of battening down the hatches. You may hope the storm misses you by but you don't leave your survival based on hope.

Much of this is about how to behave and what to do as we enter the storm, as well as having a plan B (or C, or D...) in case plan A doesn't work. It also means making some difficult choices - if you were a cargo ship in a storm, to what degree would you risk survival of the whole ship to try to preserve all of the cargo?

Finally, disaster recovery is about ensuring that you have a strong 'out of crisis or disaster' plan that means your most important faculties or critical success factors have been preserved. That means knowing what they are likely to be going into the storm, so that you make sure they aren't casualties of that storm.

An example of this might be your aspiration to be a specialist Trust focusing on the highest possible complexity of care. That is a very difficult aspiration to achieve when times change if nobody wants to work for you because of your pre- and during-storm behaviour. You need look no further than Barts Health to see this dilemma in action.

With all that said and before we get stuck in, I want to cover just two more important issues before we really start on guidance, one of which actually is the very first piece of guidance. They are:

- Understanding what HealthCRASH is and means

- Upgrading our understanding at all levels

Both of these contain keys to behaving in a manner consistent with survival and future success.

What Actually IS HealthCRASH?

Before going any further, I think it might be useful to provide a few perspectives on what HealthCRASH is and what it might look like, accepting that it will be different from place to place and nobody really knows. Consequently, these are a few possibilities and must be taken as such, not as gospel.

To understand this, I want to revisit the 'who you are' question. Disaster could take many forms and many courses, depending on your perspective. As an organisational leader, disaster may be a catastrophic failure in quality and safety, precipitating financial collapse, leading to the organisation being put into administration, with no saviours and never recovering.

We already have examples of that, with Mid Staffordshire being the most prominent. This puts organisational disaster aversion in context. If successful, the organisation may not go into administration but that does not mean it will not be touched by HealthCRASH. HealthCRASH of our system, will have effects on each organisation BUT only some will survive.

Unless Government provides that financial window of opportunity, I have a statement that I frequently make that puts HealthCRASH in perspective at an organisational level. It goes like this; *even in HealthCRASH, and as long as the true cost of demand in the way we are currently addressing it costs more than the available funding, there is no reason why any single organisation should fail but at the same time it is completely impossible for all to survive.*

There's an imperative in HealthCRASH to put yourself in the surviving category by your decisions and actions. I am saying it is as much a distinct choice - a commitment - as it is a function of circumstances. For those learning both what to do and how to do it to put themselves in the surviving category, HealthCRASH needs to be approached with respect but not necessarily fear.

It is possible for a Trust to survive but individual services not to. This is a reality already and we have a myriad of examples where services have failed to learn how to put themselves in the surviving category, typically losing out to commercial organisations that know how to do just that. To be clear, that's not back-door privatisation. It's a grass roots failure to learn how to adapt and respond to system-mediated changes. It has poor understanding, inappropriate organisational structure and culture and a massive dose of inertia at its heart.

Services (essentially all of the leaders and staff within those services) have to understand what can and might happen to them and how to respond intelligently. We know that each service is a separate 'business unit' or service-line - a core principle of service line management. However, I prefer to think of this somewhat differently.

I tend to view a Trust as a holding company. If that Trust is an Acute Trust, it will have within its organisational envelope, 40+ individual, highly complex, unique but related, multimillion pound clinical businesses. Each needs to adopt a strategic course that reflects its circumstances and the direction of travel that the system is taking in that area of care. At the same time, it needs to be in alignment with its fellow services and Trust as a whole.

This distinction is an important one. A Trust may experience adverse effects in a service and it might not threaten the Trust as a whole. However, if enough services are in trouble, then the Trust is in trouble. Trust performance is really the aggregated performances of its individual clinical businesses. It is a core reason why the move towards service-led isn't optional.

This also goes part way to explaining why a 'typical' approach by management consultants falls short of delivering meaningful improvement. For a Trust in deep trouble, a forensic analysis of the Trust-level data fails to recognise the myriad of differences between individual services. Consequently, a one-size-fits-all (or nobody) solution e.g. workforce reform and controls, tends then to have differential effects that when aggregated often mean no overall change but a tremendous amount of further damage. Sadly, I would reference Barts Health again, if you want an example.

At this point, considering HealthCRASH from the service level, it means that although we will look at what I will describe as organisational-level approaches or guidance, we are really discussing a mixture of Trust and service-level guidance. In a surviving Trust, that is built on a distributed leadership environment with the principles of service-led firmly at play.

So what might HealthCRASH mean, if you are an individual? It could mean the loss of your livelihood because a hospital is put into administration, or your individual service is lost. It could be a personal health crisis as you try to cope with overwhelming load in impossible circumstances. Aversion in this latter case will be much more about protecting yourself.

Thinking through to the other side of HealthCRASH, recovery might mean making sure you maintain your health and professional reputation so that you may seize opportunities on the other side with a largely intact life.

All of this aside, I think it is also important to spend a short, uncomfortable paragraph considering just what forms HealthCRASH might take and what that might mean. This is not to be alarmist but it is to reinforce that we are discussing a set of circumstances of the utmost severity and with very real consequences to all involved.

The Dark Side of HealthCRASH

I know of two Trusts that have come within days of not being able to run their payroll without emergency support from the system. Whereas the system may currently be able and willing to loan money (loans being a very questionable, sub-prime precipitator of HealthCRASH), this brings into reality the principle that you cannot pay for things if you have no cash. Our NHS is just as subject to that reality as anybody else.

So far, to the best of my knowledge and however close we have come, this has not yet happened. However, the minute a Trust is even a few days late with its payroll, individuals have claims against that Trust, the Trust is in breach of contract, a myriad of additional charges will need refunding to individuals, when they don't make their mortgage payments on time, along with letters of explanation from the employer and more. Essentially, stress turns into chaos and this will massively impact the day job of delivering care.

Individuals calmly go about their day job under normal circumstances, in the belief that the end of the month will produce pay, on time, for them to fulfil their commitments. The minute that belief changes to one of uncertainty, we have major behaviour problems. It would be nigh on impossible for the 'average' person to work as normal whilst remaining unsure that they are going to get paid.

As soon as we have organisations in this type of chaos (some will say 'more' chaos, reflecting how difficult some are already finding things), we will start to see the darker side of HealthCRASH emerging. What we have to some degree already will become the mainstream driver of behaviour - personal survival. This is a fight-

or-flight set of responses that reduces the chances of intelligent, rational, steady-handed measures being taken and instead pushes the organisation into a downwards spiral of limbically-driven behaviours.

It is important to realise that this is the focus of disaster preparation. How we respond at this point is crucial to whether we survive as an organisation, or sink.

As soon as we are at this point, lives are being affected and individuals will start running. Patients will find they do not have access to services when they need them and we will be in full blown HealthCRASH. This immediate withdrawal of discretionary effort and reduction in effort, along with the administrative chaos, will result in an acute decline in financial performance alongside an increase in costs. Remember this is on the back of already dire financial performance.

It also has a knock-on effect and we have to be ready and prepared for this. As we speak, Worcestershire Acute Hospitals NHS Trust is in more crisis than most. It has seen mass-resignations in its emergency care service, only just replaced. The local CCG has written to GPs advising them against referring patients for elective care. In a Trust already on the edge of financial collapse, this could be a precipitating factor. What happens next?

Whilst disaster ensues locally, patients demand their constitutional right to care and elect to go elsewhere. Where do they go? The next Trust suddenly finds themselves with rapidly increasing referrals. If it isn't careful, this precipitates a crisis here too, whether it comes operationally or financially. In either Trust, the nail in the coffin is staff who have had enough or who just can't take any more, physically or mentally. When they walk, we have a spiral that unravels across a health economy.

If you feel that I am describing the stuff of disaster movies, that's the point. Ebola was the stuff of a disaster movie. It became that because the players, individual and organisational, were not ready, did not know how to act, had no plan B and were subject to the full force of a crisis turning into a disaster. If this is scary, we had better underline that mental note to do something meaningful. NOBODY wants to see this happening but I have chosen to illustrate it with an example that is far more real than hypothetical (Worcs Acute, not Ebola).

Irrespective of perspective, I think we all have to be realistic that the days during HealthCRASH will be deeply unpleasant and worrying, nothing will seem easy and not everything will feel palatable, regardless of how necessary. The leader of that ship in a storm needs to accept that they might need to take what in calm weather would seem like extreme action.

If you are hoping for easy comfortable answers I am going to disappoint. Nobody said that leadership was easy and that takes on a whole new meaning when in the thick of something like HealthCRASH.

Rudolph Giuliani, ex-Mayor of New York, woke up one morning to find two planes parked in tall buildings. It was always going to be a terrible time but what he chose to do was crucial to an acceptable outcome downstream. If you are thinking that's a rather extreme example, I would remind you that in Mid Staffordshire, there were 1,197 unexpected deaths in circumstances that are arguably an early warning of the very scenarios I am alluding to.

What's more, that's just one Trust in a system with nearly 250 that has the potential to spiral out of control. In comparison, 3,000 people died in the Twin Towers and it resulted in a trebling of the annual Homeland Security budget in the following decade to ensure it never happened again. We might ask why 3,000 unacceptable deaths produces such profound changes but the prospect or possibility of 50 times that, with more guiding evidence already in existence, produces so little response in the right places (or any places).

With that rather knee-trembling set of thoughts in mind, we had better turn ourselves to the second issue I wanted to discuss. Swiftly. Fortunately, this is also the start of solution building.

Upgrading our Level of Understanding

I cannot stress more strongly the profound importance of this advice. Why? Because failure in this arena is already the primary root cause of the poop we are in and thus perhaps the single most important step in learning how to get ourselves back out.

I have seen so many examples of failure mediated through the stimulus-response behaviour of individuals, each with a level of responsibility alone that has the potential to cause large scale destruction within their sphere of influence. I will share some of those examples or scenarios, as it is perhaps the best way to illustrate the problem and thus the importance of the advice.

For every scenario actually shared, I could compile ten times that if you had the reading tolerance. Unfortunately, you probably do not, but fortunately, I don't actually need to. I am going to share 5 examples and they will be enough.

Firstly, let me outline the root cause problem so that you can see how the following examples occur. That problem is INSUFFICIENT UNDERSTANDING at all levels but especially in decision-makers or those asked to respond to somebody else's decisions e.g. by transforming.

It leads organisations into trying to move forward without consensus. This is virtually impossible in a system where very few people have true authority. We have highly complex professional structures and if we ignore this, or try to go round this, we fall foul of its strength. That strength was built in for good reason. Somebody needed to advocate for the patient over and above every other consideration.

However, the 'not in the patient's best interest, get out of jail free card' is now very much an Achilles Heel in times of transformation because it prevents organisations from 'just doing it'.

That is not to say we should be disbanding that ethical defence structure - far from it. I believe we need it more today than ever before. We already have a growing list of failures and scandals even with it, let alone without it.

I am saying that we are trying to upgrade our system but without having upgraded our thinking and understanding. In the absence of that vital thinking and understanding, we cannot reach consensus and without consensus in a system where we have little explicit authority, we cannot lead any significant change. We are trapped by the singular issue alone of insufficient and inconsistent understanding.

What makes it worse is that our response to this difficulty is not to fix the root cause but to do things without consensus or do things where we have all drawn the wrong conclusion, collectively, because ALL of our understanding is inadequate. I see both, almost daily. My examples are just a small illustration of a massive, enduring problem.

The reason I am stressing this so strongly is that if this has contributed from us going from stability to the edge of HealthCRASH, then whilst in HealthCRASH it has to ability to even more rapidly unfold a crisis into a disaster. Let's look at those scenarios.

E1 - Protecting What You Shouldn't

Arguably, this is not a specific example but an example of a specific repeated behaviour that I have seen over and over again. Lord Darzi indicated a number of changes to the locus of care, determined by its complexity, diagnostic and treatment predictability, its diagnostic and treatment difficulty and even its volume.

These changes to locus of care were to address the core issue that we still had our largely 1948 system but care options, patient population and disease burden had shifted massively. Essentially, we had innovated in medicine but not in delivery model and we were now struggling with a significant mismatch that was only going to get worse with an aging population.

Examples of these locus changes included moving simple, routine care into primary care locations, physically closer to patients and into simpler, cheaper delivery models, volume procedures into treatment centres and complex care into fewer but larger tertiary organisations. Across the board, we have seen large scale resistance to this.

Tertiary centres have sought to hang on to too much routine care, leaving them with insufficient capacity to take more complex care and at the same time, smaller centres have hung onto some complex care because it is interesting. More commonly, DGHs have tried to hang onto simple care that is destined for community locations, often citing that they need it for organisational financial stability.

You have failed understanding at play across multiple levels of hierarchy. Firstly, everybody fails to understand they are engaging in something futile. The system has been adapted to see these changes happen regardless of whether providers want them to, with the emergence of Any Qualified Provider, changed local commissioning and even organically by influencing the expectations of patients. If you aren't meant to hang on to it, you can't hang on to it for long unless you adapt your model!

Trusts and services spend far more time justifying why, for instance, community is the wrong place to run a routine service, than thinking about how to design a community-based service in alignment with the system's direction of travel, which we have known since Lord Darzi! Services out of alignment with the system will fail. But, they will not end up in alignment with the system if they do not understand the system.

E2 - Ignoring the New Specification

With the same dysfunctional underpinning, I see tender after tender lost to commercial or other organisations because the existing 'contract holder' fails to match up to the tender specification. Why? Because it represents a change of delivery model.

Instead, they fall into the trap of trying to persuade those running the tender that their specification is 'better' somehow than the one being used to tender. Often this is both a failure to understand why the tender is being run in the first place and a failure to appreciate how little influence an existing provider necessarily has for certain types of things (let alone a failure to know how to win tenders).

E3 - Seeing Things Simplistically

My example here goes to the heart of our financial woes at a provider level. It will hit a chord with many. We have engaged in a number of simplistic responses to complex problems. These simplistic responses then create new problems, leading to further woe. We respond to these simplistically too. We are constantly moving away from stability.

I am now challenged with conveying a complex problem in a simple enough way to make it understandable, but here goes...

In response to austerity and the emergence of deficits, a number of our responses have been simplistic (and ill thought through). We have reduced staffing and closed wards to save money. But, that already fails to consider we have increasing demand.

We have also failed to recognise that we have far more widely fluctuating demand, partly due to demand increases, partly due to choice and partly due to the removal of many organisational boundaries or catchment areas and yet we continue to run fixed capacity organisations.

We have also failed to understand the importance of marginal rates (receiving less money for a type of care if our activity levels increase over certain historic thresholds). This has been most significant with emergency care, which has risen significantly and until recently carried a marginal rate of only 30% of the national tariff.

So how has this played out? Our emergency care activity has gone up whilst our overall capacity has come down (without getting into social care challenges and other confounding factors). In our fixed, insufficient capacity organisations, given we can't turn off the emergency care tap easily, this additional work <u>at a marginal rate</u> displaces elective work at the full rate.

The effect of this is to result in an organisation doing the same amount of work on the same level of resource but receiving less money and thus proceeding to develop a deficit. The increase in emergency may even require agency staff to cope with, resulting in higher costs too, on less money.

I would argue that the marginal rate (itself evidence of a system that can't afford to cover the full cost of demand) is only part of the problem. Inappropriate reductions in beds, staffing, the failure to develop flexible capacity, the failure to find ways to protect elective case load and more are part of the problem too.

To illustrate just how much simplistic thinking is involved, the response to a larger deficit caused by this scenario is frequently to try to save more money through means that further reduce capacity. That vicious cycle makes matters worse and is a major contributor to the issues we face today.

Let's be clear though; this is a problem mediated through simplistic thinking, poor understanding and regulator behaviour too. Yes, poor understanding exists at ALL levels, not just within Trusts.

E4 - Behaving with Authority

If the last example was alive and well across the acute sector, then this is literally endemic from top to bottom. It starts with the false assumption of authority, often bestowed with a grand job title like Director of Something or Chief Executive of Somewhere.

I will say straight out that you almost certainly don't have true authority and even if you have immediate authority, those you instruct probably do not have enough authority to carry the instructions on down the organisation or system. And yet so many are almost certainly behaving as if they do, causing large scale destruction to the internal, collaborative working relationships and trust. This is a crucial issue to survival.

This is also a complex problem in its own right and it has poor understanding and thinking both at play. Let's say you are a Strategy Director of an Acute Trust and you recognise you need to adapt your dermatology service to a partly hospital, partly community-based model, very consistent with the system direction of travel. So, you go and speak with the Dermatologists, a long standing group of senior consultants with a career in hospital medicine. You discuss those plans.

However, they don't fully understand the system and try to persuade you that the service will be cheaper, more efficient and certainly higher quality if maintained in hospital. They point out that it will take more staff to run the community model and we are already under cost-pressures.

As a group, they are failing to understand the system direction of travel AND how much power they (the Trust) have. On the other hand, you have very little ability to 'tell' them to adapt and they know they can slow that process down almost 'forever' if they don't engage because you have little ability to move them and they haven't done anything wrong. You can't simply replace them.

So how does this play out. You and the Trust become more and more stressed at the vulnerability of your dermatology service but the dermatologists see your heightened attempts to introduce reason and stronger persuasion as examples of your own failure to understand what constitutes best care and of bullying and coercion, which they should resist still further.

Then, a tender is run by the commissioners for a community-based dermatology service and your Trust is wholly behind where it needs to be in terms of tender readiness. It loses, and everybody blames everybody else and the system and the circumstances. If I had a pound for every time a version of this had played out...

The reality is that there was a failure to understand the system, the direction of travel, behaviour, change, leadership and what produces security and ALL parties were culpable to some degree. Ironically, it often takes the loss of a service for the players to understand what can happen and even then, they will find reasons to justify why it wasn't their fault.

It should be recognised here that the Strategy Director didn't try to exert the degree of authority that I see being exerted in many Trusts. We have lots of examples of outright bullying (and sorry, Barts Health is again a prominent example). However, he or she did fail to understand how to lead change when you don't have authority and that is very much part of the challenges we face.

E5 - Failing to Seize Opportunity

The final scenario is again endemic and illustrates a difference in ethos between the commercial sector and NHS organisations. To characterise that difference, the commercial sector is nimble and focused on seeking out opportunities and the NHS tends to be slow to decide, slow moving and spends most of its time looking over its shoulder (and even then, not adequately).

The consequence of this is that as long as we have a competitive system, the NHS will tend to lose out to commercial competition. This was illustrated beyond reasonable doubt by an evaluation in 2013 of 57 consecutive tenders under Any Qualified Provider, 39 of which went to the commercial sector.

At the time, this brought hails of vitriol over the privatisation of the NHS and yet I was far more inclined to think of this as a nearly total failure to understand how the system was changing, what it took to be successful in the new system and then develop those capabilities and tendencies. The system has changed but the existing organisations have not upgraded their thinking and behaviour to remain successful in that system. That is always going to turn out badly for the existing players.

I have previously made the statement that we live in an era where there has never been more opportunity but at the same time, never more threat. The NHS orientates to defending itself against threat (mostly too late and in the wrong way) but without the same attention to seizing opportunity. That leaves it vulnerable to loss but without the compensating gains. You could say that it is hell bent on staying the same by protecting what it has in a system that is more about change.

As a very direct example, I know of one Trust presented with a business case by a service to build a sports medicine service that would have added considerable net income to the bottom line. The Trust already had the necessary gym and sports facilities on its campus, largely unused for healthcare purposes, so there wasn't a requirement for significant capital investment. The demand had been analysed and was real. However, there was the need for some investment and the business case got rejected.

This was about as certain an opportunity as you are ever likely to find in a business environment. However, this Trust was strongly orientated towards the status quo, far more interested in CIP and continues to have what appears to be an immovable deficit. That will probably always be the case, with those behaviours, backed by that attitude or orientation.

It's a failure to upgrade the thinking. I am inclined to think they may recognise themselves from the example. I am guessing that denial will also come into play, probably along the justification lines of 'not having the cash' even if they wanted to approve it. Well, that's a failure to understand how to leverage cash - another example of outdated thinking or understanding. Do you think Mr Branson always uses his own money for his next venture?

A Critical Need

We have to be explicitly clear here on both the root cause of the problem and the suggested solution. This is a function of both insufficient or poor understanding and inappropriate or poor thinking. These are different aspects of the same problem. Both are at play.

It cannot have escaped your notice that many of our problems, as we face them today within our organisations, are functions of this failure playing out across repeated decisions, actions and interactions over time. If we are to survive HealthCRASH and thrive on the other side, this has to be our number one priority - never being this cognitively vulnerable again.

We need a wholly different level of understanding and it needs to exist from top to bottom in our organisations and certainly in us as individuals. Every day 'something' happens that requires a response. How that turns out for us depends on our response. Our response depends on our level of understanding, how shared that understanding is and thus, our ability to reach <u>consensus</u> on the genuinely <u>best choice</u> of course of action.

As illustrated by the strategic change in dermatology, if we are working off a poor or partial picture of the way things work today, in already horribly difficult circumstances, it leads us to inadvertently take the wrong road. If we all understand something differently, we struggle to reach consensus and that lack of consensus turns into inertia or 'stay the same' when change might be necessary for survival.

If this is problematic now, it takes on a whole new level of importance through HealthCRASH. The stakes will be higher, the policies more erratic, the changes more frequent and the consequences more grave. Our ability to respond intelligently and cohesively will perhaps be the single biggest determinant of our likelihood of emerging securely on the other side.

There's another component - the thinking. To be more specific, this is a combination of learning how to THINK most appropriately in spite of our FEELINGS. This is a big ask on my part but an important one. When we develop a negative, emotional response, it turns off our ability to think logically, rationally and calmly. Instead, we either deny or disengage (flight) or justify and defend (more of a fight response).

This goes to the heart of disaster preparation - the ability to think clearly in circumstances that are positively demanding a limbic response. This requires very specific preparation. In organisations that have not undergone this, as pressure increases they will likely unravel much faster than the average, making recovery far less likely.

If we examine our dermatologists, we can see this alive and not well. It would be easy to judge their response as purely on the basis that they didn't appreciate how the system was changing and where risk and threat was to be found. However, even when presented with that reality by people who did, their response was to misjudge the motivation or intention (Trust bullying, rather than concern for service loss).

That error turned out to be a fatal error of judgement. Whereas poor understanding of how the system works, along with who is able to do what and how, were undoubtedly contributing factors, almost certainly beliefs, values and ideological challenge were at play too. This was a group of individuals blind to their own blind spots and mental processing, with a limbic response triggered unfortunately by the Strategy Director, who started in wholly the wrong place to carry this change.

As for the dermatologists, to what degree was their judgement of the appropriateness of a mixed hospital-community model influenced by their historical knowledge and experience of the structure of dermatology? How much was their judgement of its acceptability underpinned by rationale, objective thought versus what this means to them as <u>hospital</u> specialists?

Once a thought process such as "this is a threat to the professional structure of dermatology" creeps in, it starts to turn off a more detached, objective examination of the unfolding scenario. In effect, all subsequent circumstances get moulded and interpreted by the pre-existing mental models and a good dose of limbic processing. None of this helps in producing a response grounded in the best interests of the service and Trust.

We are likely to be entering a period involving a heightened pace of change but with the continued existence of a myriad of policies that already don't fit together very well. A successful outcome for Trusts and services will mean exercising the very best of judgement, underpinned by a deep understanding of how things work.

It is important in all that HealthCRASH is likely to bring in adverse behaviours and circumstances to appreciate that the existing policies and processes may not all change. We will most likely be working in an environment where mad, panic-driven things are happening around us and yet we will still be subject to the constraints of the existing policies.

Success will depend on understanding them, knowing their effects and likelihood of happening and in keeping up-to-date with what is actually changing and how. It will also come from thinking through how to act when the policies and your best interests seem at odds with each other, whilst being certain about what is real versus what might be a function of your own limbic processing. THAT is going to require upgraded thinking of the highest level. I can put it no more strongly.

I want to reiterate that having the right thinking and judgement is necessary for two key reasons, both linking directly to your survival - coming up with the right response and reaching consensus on that to a sufficient degree that a group is prepared to act on it. This means that it isn't sufficient for a few to have this understanding, it must be embedded in everybody.

Finally, at an organisational level, although it introduces us to the personal level very nicely, an absence of this thinking and understanding leaves us like a rabbit caught in the headlights when faced with a rapidly oncoming truck or the like (change, challenge, curveball, tender...), at a time when decision and action are paramount. We all know what happens to that rabbit.

The Individual Component

Having laid out how important good judgement is to service security, I want to spend a moment or two on how important it is for individuals i.e. you! Every day you are faced with needing to exercise good judgement, which is itself dependent on the dual components of depth of understanding and mastery of thinking, including how to control for the likelihood of limbic processing.

What should you support? What should you resist? How will you ensure good thinking around you? How will you influence decisions and strategies? How will you know when the wrong things are happening?

Many will by now have the direct experience of knowing they resisted something that perhaps they shouldn't have, or supported a decision that should have been different, or disengaged from an issue that was of crucial importance. What sorts out the leaders from the 'also ran' is the ability to accept you got it wrong (it's OK, we're human, it's not a character flaw) and to seek out and recognise why. In many cases, the issue will lie in something you needed to know but didn't, along with how you thought about it.

I am guessing that at the point of the decision, you were not even conscious of how you were thinking and what was causing the specific emotions you had. You went with 'gut feel' perhaps later rationalised with some consistent reasoning. The problem is that you would only have been seeking reasoning or evidence that supported your already determined position, not that produced inconvenient inconsistencies. Our ability to control for this behavioural tendency is crucial to our effectiveness as leaders and survival as individuals.

Depth of understanding is crucial to your own decisions and actions. Many will find themselves in organisations that will not survive, as I have already alluded to. Your personal security is based on knowing to what degree an organisation is adopting the right approaches versus taking a course of action likely to precipitate its own demise. Whereas some of that can be assessed intuitively and is more obvious, some of it will require a deep level of understanding.

Let me ask you this; if you absolutely knew your organisation was taking a course of action that would result in its likely demise and it wouldn't change this despite your best attempts, to what degree would you be willing to put your own health, well-being and reputation on the line regardless?

You see, your decisions are inextricably linked to what you know and how you think. You owe it to yourself to upgrade this and especially as we enter a period where how you think will be so crucial to how it turns out for you.

My personal view is that had this been recognised (or listened to) many years ago, we could have avoided much of the adversity we are now facing. However, now that we are facing an increasing level of adversity, it is totally vital that we aren't personally contributing further to it through our own partial views and superficial level of insight. Our own survival is dependent on it too.

Organisational Responses & Guidance

We are going to look at these through the three concurrent phases, of aversion, preparation and recovery. This chapter is aimed firmly at Boards, executive and non-executive, senior managers, GP Principals, Practice Managers and leaders of clinical services, including clinical leads, matrons and managers, along with the myriad of other leaders across the different structures we have in play across healthcare organisations.

Before we go any further, I want to clarify something. IF you have concluded (and I guess that you have, given you are still reading) that HealthCRASH is a probability, if not a certainty, then we are IN a crisis. The point is, we are already in that crisis. Without responding to that crisis, we run the risk of it turning into a disaster, for us. Because we don't operate in a vacuum, however well we try to prevent this, a disaster may unfold.

I am explaining this because we need to know what our 3 concurrent phases are really about. In understanding that, we stand the best chances of doing enough of the right things.

Disaster Aversion is about not turning a crisis into a disaster, by recognising the signs and symptoms, steadily turning back around and making our way back to stability.

Disaster Preparation is about accepting the possibility in such severe circumstances that it may affect us adversely and significantly enough that we may not survive unless we know what to do. Yes, some of this is about preventing a 'late stage' or 'fast moving' crisis turning into a disaster but much is also about how to behave and what to do when finding yourself with a disaster on your hands. That section deals with both.

Disaster Recovery is about rebuilding yourself. Whereas it might seem that this is an 'after the event' activity, strong organisations recognising the potential for a disaster, plan for this from the start, so that they know what to hang on to and what to let go of to leave themselves in the best survival state.

It is worth recognising that leaders are human. Consequently, although this section is encouraging a steady-handed approach to preparation and passage through, we all have to be mindful that leaders are as subject to maladaptive responses and limbic behaviour as anybody else. We look to our leaders for strength in times of crisis but we need to recognise the need to look after them too.

Whereas finding ourselves in a sinking ship tends to foster a shared sense of purpose, finding ourselves in a sinking organisation will frequently precipitate the leaders bailing first, something we are seeing happen at an alarming rate. We have to understand this is part of the problem. We need stability.

Finally, before delving into the advice itself, I want to reiterate that the purpose of this book was never to provide a granular blueprint. To provide one, I would be both naïve and arrogant. We have enough of that already and I would suggest it has been an enduring part of the problems we have - for an individual or group to believe that, when facing all of that complexity, they have THE answer. We call it the God Complex and I do not want to be a participant. There's too much at stake.

Instead, I am going to try to provide a set of principles on how to think and act, along with some more specific guidance that is largely proven i.e. no longer a guess.

There is a surprising body of evidence on disaster preparation, mitigation and recovery but sadly I see very little of it being brought into play. Let's hope we can change that.

There is an even bigger body of evidence around behaviour, and I have been tapping into that throughout the book. Some of the understanding, from an organisational perspective, is really quite new (especially how bits fit together) and comparatively little from a healthcare environment specifically.

However, unless we think that our healthcare people are fundamentally different to, rather than a somewhat unique subset of 'people' then the work is important. I do hope you won't fall into the trap of thinking that somehow healthcare professionals have a different set of neurological plumbing to others and thus deny the relevance and importance of what I am about to unfold.

Disaster Aversion

Ironically, despite the level of difficulty we find ourselves in, there is a huge amount you can do as a service or organisational leader to mitigate the effects of HealthCRASH. However, I feel compelled to express ongoing, huge frustration that organisations have resolutely failed to engage in much, if any of it, in favour of towing the NHSE/ regulator party line. I am going to be very harsh and ask; how well has that turned out for you?

What I am NOT going to recommend is 'getting a grip', given that much of the mess we are in is as a direct result of just such action. Disaster aversion for organisations is about building organisational resilience generally and specifically in factors that are critical to survival and success. We need to understand what these critical factors are and thus what to do to preserve them or install them if they are absent.

Rapid Adaptability

If a crisis is characterised by anything, it is how rapidly circumstances change. In circumstances that might change very rapidly, often with severe, adverse consequences if they do, rapid adaptability is by far the most important capability to have. We need to be clear though, this is rapid adaptability and not limbic reactivity, which tends to get you into even more hot water.

Returning to our Leadership Potency Framework, rapid adaptability comes from picking up early WHETHER something needs solving, addressing or changing and then developing a considered response of the right urgency and magnitude (WHAT) in a manner that maximises its chances of happening (HOW). The good news is that what builds rapid adaptability is also consistent with resilience in many of the other critical success factors.

The core challenge we (you) face is that the organisational structure and control processes we operate, especially in Hospital Trusts, are at complete odds with rapid adaptability, or indeed Leadership Potency. Besides this alone being perhaps the biggest predictor that you will not survive, it tends to result in a level of clinical-managerial divide and demoralised staff that is wholly inconsistent with anything rapid actually happening. I suspect I don't have to persuade you of that. Just look around you.

What's more, those same staff are not going to be prepared to go to the ends of the earth to save you when there is no shared sense of purpose or responsibility. They are likely to view your preceding actions as having nothing but negative impacts on them and their ability to preserve patient care. The Trust becomes THEM versus US, the point being that it is no longer cohesive.

This results in you being part of the problem and thus no real reason to dig so much deeper to help save you. As if that weren't enough, this structure and way of working is wholly inconsistent with rapidly generating intelligent solutions and responses to what are genuinely complex circumstances.

It has to change and very fast indeed. This should be your number 1 aversion priority because it will kill you if you don't and yet provides you with many of the answers if you do.

But change how and to what?

The Service-led Organisation

The answer is transformation towards the clinically-led or service-led organisation. This is a change in structure, behaviour, decision-making and governance, resulting in a distributed leadership approach across an organisation of semi-independent, multimillion pound clinical businesses.

If you are thinking this takes years and is fraught with traps, I will agree with you in so far as that being true if you approach it the wrong way with insufficient support. I will openly say or admit though that it is more 'comfortable' taking years but given the reality that you don't have years, I am going to encourage you to 'get over it' and learn the right way, fast. You may well feel you can't afford to do it swiftly and I am going to say you can't afford not to.

If you have any lingering doubt about the necessity or advisability of this, I would remind you of the preceding chapter on how to approach HealthCRASH, prior to us getting into this specific advice. You may recall that a big part of the reason you are where you are is because you have failed to gain traction on transformation. That is absolutely because you do not carry sufficient authority and you do not have the structural and cultural conditions for it to happen otherwise. The service-led organisation is about creating that ability to adapt swiftly and intelligently.

The point is that the service-led organisation is one with a collection of services, where each has robust leadership potency and consequently, rapid adaptability. However, it is vital to appreciate that this structural change needs to be accompanied by a disbanding of control mechanisms in favour of each service having the freedom to operate and adapt, along with a strong, shared sense of responsibility that comes with that freedom. We are talking about a move to a trust-based environment where rapid adaptability of the whole is underpinned by the freer flowing nature of the parts.

What is abundantly clear is that this is a very complex change, even if it doesn't have to be a long one. It requires a common basis for decision-making and a shared understanding of what's expected and what's not, along with how to deal with issues occurring in different levels of the organisation.

A significant change difficulty is that the existing control structures are presided over by individuals who go from having significant control, authority and status, to being service providers to the very people they might perhaps have viewed as resisters and dissenters before. This group has the ability to undermine this transition and I have seen first-hand how they can sabotage the very change on which their security is truly built. The role of the executive team is crucial in controlling for this.

I am frequently struck by just how many say they are moving towards service-led but how few come even close to having the right pieces in place. They view it as a technical and structural change and it is almost entirely a complex behavioural change, in which structure and process are just necessary enabling parts. I am saying that many aspire to it and virtually nobody does what they need to do to ensure it happens.

Ironically, I have seen organisations start down this road, with all of the above failings, and consequently fail to see the real effect shine through, to then pull back and conclude that service-led isn't the answer. Apart from conveniently forgetting that Trust-led didn't produce any greater benefit, they are confusing 'calling' their organisation service-led with genuinely 'being' service-led.

In effect, that's the equivalent of sticking a Ferrari badge on a Kia and expecting it to go from 0 - 60 in under 4 seconds. If you want different performance you have to build a different engine (and chassis - the structural change to support it). You don't get there by saying "we can afford to move the badge over but not so sure we can afford those other expensive parts".

A repeated problem emerging from this behaviour is that Boards then convince the regulators that they are 'doing this' as part of improving performance. That disappoints everybody because the underlying reality is no change. It is very much time to recognise what is necessary to achieve this most important of changes. Your survival depends on it. Please take it seriously.

I am sure that the naysayers, deniers and defensive-reasoners will find it easy to discount the above perspective. That's OK, it's your choice, but before you discount it completely, also consider this.

You have almost certainly spent much of the last few years creating the near-perfect conditions for staff rebellion and transformation resistance. You have almost certainly failed in true ENABLEMENT. Are you seriously expecting a miraculous transformation to service-led without adequate enablement?

If the mean level of understanding of what's happening in our system and why, was just 4.8 out of 20 (our research, discussed already), across the consultant body, that's already wholly inconsistent with developing the necessary level of WILL for this change to happen. Even with WILL, those same individuals have no spare CAPACITY, let alone the SKILL - knowledge, skills and insight - to know what to do, hence the previous chapter. Even if you get this far, the majority of organisations then continue to lead those service leaders <u>with</u> AUTHORITY, rather than vest in them the true authority they need.

Instead, you continue to lead them as though you <u>have</u> AUTHORITY over them, when in fact you do not and especially not clinical ones, on whom you rely to deliver the organisational purpose. You cannot succeed without their buy in and you cannot get that buy in when they do not understand.

Uncomfortable though it is to accept, you will only create organisational resilience, stability and rapid flexibility if you create intelligently designed solutions that are acceptable and understood by those clinical teams because only when you and they are in consensus will you get meaningful and rapid action. However, to gain that level of acceptance for plans and strategies, the people that need to implement will need to have developed them i.e. they need to be service-led.

Additionally, given that HealthCRASH will unfold differently in various specialties, many of those meaningful solutions and strategies will need to be service-specific and I seriously doubt you have the depth of clinical expertise or the leadership capacity in the centre to produce enough intelligent and acceptable solutions that are genuinely grounded in the reality facing each individual service. Without that, you will continue to face intransigence and insurmountable resistance.

Those strategies and solutions need to come from the services themselves, generated and implemented by a group of people with a MUCH higher level of thinking, capability and capacity than they currently have. And that's why you need 'service-led' as a necessity, not an option.

Vital Clinical Mitigation

My next piece of aversion or mitigation advice, is one that is controversial. It has produced more denial and defensiveness than I care to reflect on and yet ironically, has the potential to create much of that vital window we so desperately need. What's more, it 'should' be acceptable to everybody, given that it relies on producing significant clinical and financial improvement hand in hand. What's not to love?

I am referring to a body of clinical improvement work that has the ability to radically transform both quality and financial footprint if seized appropriately. You would think that this is a no-brainer in a system crying out for answers. What's more, it's not even a maybe, because the designer of the work has utilised it on his own service and transformed the clinical, financial and operational performance, including a massive, swift, permanent reduction in the required bed base.

His ongoing analyses demonstrate that there are very few services that it doesn't apply to and that its overall potential alone could reset the financial balance, at least for the time being. However, despite this potential, the body of work meets with considerable resistance, denial and open defensiveness, both from clinical services and organisationally.

I am hoping by now that you are at least comfortable with the idea that I am not easily misled. In a book titled HealthCRASH, providing advice designed for some of our darkest times, this is not something I am going to raise without being sure.

What's more, this form of clinical improvement is designed to tackle the growing mismatch between our current delivery models and the complex needs of an ageing, increasingly frail population. We have to realise that some of our deepest flow issues, system-wide, exist because of this mismatch. This goes to the heart of the unsustainability of our healthcare system and provides real answers.

The potential is unquestionably real but the effect of such pushback, despite being devoid of other meaningful options, has been so great that it has lead the designer (and myself) to conclude that persuading individuals, services and Trusts is a futile exercise. Consequently, he (and I) took the decision to only share it with or help those prepared to give sufficient time to properly and fully understand it, with egos and preconceptions left firmly at the door.

If you are prepared to come to us and convince us that you really want to know, then we will be only too happy to share. You know where we are.

I am sure that this 'not quite advice' will cause a certain level of frustration. Why can't I just tell you what it is? Well, perhaps it's my own behavioural block but we both agree that there is no point in wasting words and breath with individuals and organisations that show such a propensity to discount what they don't understand (without wanting to dig deeper to understand it), whilst asking to be bailed because they have no other meaningful options. When you learn to be better than that, we'll be more than glad to help.

Apologies for the soapbox!

My final piece of advice could well sit in preparation as much as aversion. I am putting it in aversion because I think it needs time, debate and some detailed planning. It is going to be uncomfortable and the very advice itself has the potential, if not used appropriately, to precipitate disaster.

As I explained how HealthCRASH might look, I unfolded a scenario whereby the payroll was late. Although this was hypothetical, you will recall that I know two Trusts who have come days away from this being a reality.

The sequence of events that I articulated from there was a best guess at how it might unfold, not a worst case scenario. I see a high enough probability that this could be a true disaster-releasing event in its own right. An event that has patient care, lives, staff livelihoods and more at stake.

I don't think I would be mis-describing it as 'all hell breaking loose'. Its effects are a complex spiral of behavioural, emotional, limbic-driven actions and reactions that would most likely be unrecoverable in that worst case. At that point, what was a crisis would become a disaster, as the crisis took charge beyond what you could reasonably do to control it.

Consequently, and consistent with 'hope for the best but plan for the worst', this needs a plan. Quite what that plan is, I am struggling to feel qualified to comment but as a Director myself, I know how I would 'think' about it. And I'd think about it ahead of having to act! The last thing I'd want to be doing is making snap decisions without sufficient ability to understand their impacts and longer term outcomes.

I'd look at everything I spent money on and divide it into three distinct categories, accepting that they won't be perfect and there will be overlap. They'd be:

- Direct clinical care

- Disaster preventing
- Other stuff

As a healthcare organisation, the last thing I want to do is undermine the quality, safety and delivery efficiency of my core purpose - healthcare. My reputation is built on that and if I cease to do that well, there is no reason why anybody would want to see me survive.

Disaster-preventing spend would include things like the payroll, accepting that some is clinical and some isn't. However, given its panic-inducing potential, I'd view it as a single item at this point.

Other stuff is a more complicated category. It might contain, for instance, my expenditure around reducing carbon emissions, or money that supports revalidation. There will be a whole heap of money for training, including study-leave budgets and the myriad of programmes under way, including mandatory training. This category is my emergency fund and I would probably preserve the other two at the expense of this.

Within this category though, I need to be intelligent. For instance, perhaps some of my training spend is on upgrading the thinking and disaster preparation. I could cancel this to utilise the cash for payroll but I might be leaping out of the frying pan into the fire. Remember, preventing panic and chaos is only useful if it is part of longer term survival.

Consequently, I'd look at all of the items within this category and I'd rate them both by importance to my survival and future, as well as by the urgency with which they needed addressing. For instance, just to be controversial, if my doctors are all broadly up-to-date with revalidation, I could park ongoing activity at least for a period of time. I am not saying you should, I am saying you could. In reality, you will find a myriad of expenses that are perhaps far less important.

I think it is important to appreciate the principle here. Firstly, I am suggesting we need a plan to ensure that we can always run the payroll. That plan needs evaluating for consequences but from the context of being in a crisis, trying to prevent it becoming a disaster. Every item of spend will seem important. I am saying that some of those items become rather irrelevant if you undermine survival by continuing to support them.

I want to remind you of my previous assertion that something that might seem extreme in calm weather might be necessary in the thick of a crisis. It's the equivalent of working out which cargo to jettison to keep your boat afloat in a storm. Saving a cargo temporarily before the ship sinks just doesn't feel like the right approach if you could prevent the ship sinking by jettisoning the cargo. The key is knowing which cargo to jettison and which to save. Nothing will seem perfect but you need to have an 'eyes open' plan.

Part of this plan will be the establishment of trigger points. That a Trust could come within days of not running its payroll is a sign of two things: trust that the system will come up with the goods (on time - my bigger concern in a crisis) and no plan B when clearly one is warranted. I am sure a bunch of people sighed with relief when it all worked out. That's not a proactive plan.

I'd have or establish a level of cash I wouldn't want to go below before kicking into action my disaster aversion plan. I'd be monitoring the situation, with real data, honesty and zero denial. I'd have a trigger point for going to the system players, Monitor or the TDA, with cap in hand and a trigger point for stopping paying certain items, starting with those of least consequences and in which I can catch up later, assuming I survive.

Conscious that we are in uncharted territory, I wouldn't ignore the possibility that what you are doing comes out internally. That will have its own set of consequences and I'd approach these proactively too. That leads me neatly to disaster preparation.

Disaster Preparation

If disaster aversion is about doing as much as you can to ensure safe passage through a crisis, then disaster preparation is in part a plan B born out of the assumption that plan A probably won't be enough, given that a crisis is so unpredictable. You can never know or predict all that you need to and you cannot always control for the behaviour of others. When disaster crews responded to the first plane hitting a tower, who would have predicted a second plane, or the collapse of the towers in entirety?

Under these circumstances, decisions in the moment become much more important and often represent tipping points. It's in these moments that we most need to have our wits about us and know what to do. We know this in healthcare intuitively. It's the backbone of successful emergency or intensive care medicine at the upper end of severity.

We know that preparing people for those moments is crucial because it's not a time to be reliant on predominantly guessing or learning on the job. In part that is because we don't always know what will happen next but we do know if don't do anything it will probably turn out badly. We need a best guess, rapid assessment of its impact and a second best guess to follow it up if the first one isn't doing the job. That comes from training and experience. I am pretty sure very few will have experienced a crashing healthcare system and so we had better focus more on active preparation and training.

Mental Preparation

Without question, the single most important part of organisational disaster preparation is in addressing staff mental readiness. The research is explicit. Faced with a fast-moving crisis, only around 20% of staff have intact cognition and emotional intelligence, meaning that without the combination of mental preparation AND a plan, up to 80% of staff will act in what is referred to as a maladaptive manner.

That means that what they might do is inadvertently make matters worse. If that isn't worrying enough, the literature also reports a consistent 2% that engage in psychotic behaviour and they have the potential to sabotage, deliberately sometimes, the survival of the group. More commonly is panic-induced, uncontrolled behaviour which produces more of the same in others.

What you need from the group at this time is a concerted and coordinated response i.e. optimal individual and group thinking and behaviour. That doesn't come without distinct preparation and so that is critical step 1.

A good way of thinking about that preparation is to use the analogy of breaking bad news to a patient. Individuals are trained to expect a series of responses, not all of which are pleasant or benign. Some patients will cry, some will withdraw and some may get angry, with you. Feeling attacked by someone, especially unjustly, produces a fight or flight response in us... except when we are prepared and expect it. And that's the point. We can negate much of the adverse consequences of limbic processes by managing expectations.

There's an important second part to this that can't be ignored. We don't want to engage in the cognitive equivalent of saying "don't panic, it's what we expected" as you hit an iceberg, "but we have no clue what to do". We need mental preparation AND a plan. More importantly, the people need to know we have a plan so that they don't have to worry whether we have a plan.

I am guessing that very few of you have a plan? So, my advice is that we had better put that one on the 'to do' list and fairly near the top.

If the people need to be ready, the leaders need to be more so. Not only are they human, with the same needs as everybody else, but people will turn to them and expect guidance. There's nothing more panic-inducing than turning to your trusted leader only to hear "I've got nothing".

Returning to who responds how, ideally our crisis leaders are selected, ahead of time, from the pool of people most likely to remain calm, steady-handed and high thinking in the crisis. Each of them needs distinct responsibilities so that they act as a well-organised and cohesive leadership team.

They are going to have a common set of responsibilities that it is worth outlining, so that we better understand leader preparation. These responsibilities include:

- A distinct responsibility for something

- Understanding of the organisational plan, so that they can confidently convey a sense of control, despite a crisis

- People to guide and look after

- Finding productive jobs for those with sufficiently intact cognition

- Watching for and dealing with the adverse behaviours of those prone to limbic or psychotic behaviours

- Reporting requirements so that the disaster coordinators keep a sense of what's happening in their organisation

- Watching for adverse trigger points - signs that we are losing control

The core difference between a crisis and a disaster is that a crisis heralds the potential for damage whereas a disaster indicates the likelihood of damage, potentially unrecoverable damage. Leaders need to understand how to act intelligently in both circumstances.

Crisis leadership is about preventing it becoming a disaster and is typically characterised as steady-handed activity to systematically reduce vulnerability. Disaster leadership is much more about rapid action to prevent damage or further damage. Leaders need to know when one switches to the other and what to do in each case.

Crucial in all of this is the responsibility to look after the emotional well-being and resilience of the team. Looked after, they will see you through a crisis or disaster. If your leaders don't know how to look after them and what they need, those very same people become inadvertently disaster-precipitating.

This book cannot possibly provide the depth of insight necessary to ensure that leaders are prepared. However, I have tried to signpost you to the core areas for consideration and preparation. Disaster preparation happens ahead of time and is an active process, not a passive one.

My guess is that your leaders have probably not had crisis and disaster leadership training. If that's the case, I am suggesting you chalk it up on that 'to do' list again. After all, what's the alternative - leaving their behaviour and responses to chance, in the height of scary circumstances that they have not encountered before?

Organisational Readiness Plan

The lion's share of the remaining preparation focuses on what to do in a crisis and/ or a disaster. It's all very well having 'ready' people but ready to do what. Action is required, sensible action that is designed to ensure you emerge the other side.

There is no specific form that this should take but it needs to be clear, explicit and focus on present actions. However, those actions must also consistent with a successful future. It's not all about now.

Might I suggest approaching this as you would a serious untoward incident, in many respects? Firstly, I am assuming you have a plan for how to behave in a Serious Untoward Incident (SUI)? Exactly, it's already a crisis and possibly a disaster. It's sufficiently important that NHS England has devoted time to a generic plan and even a set of principles, illustrated in figure 19.

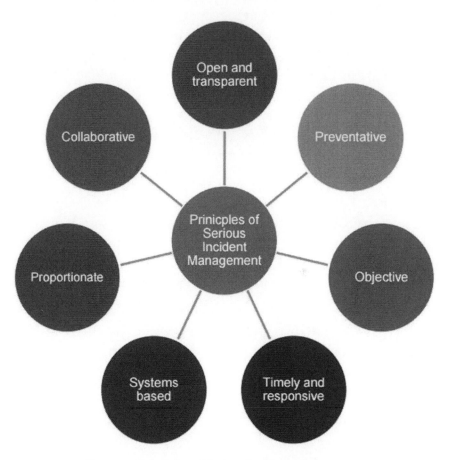

Figure 19. Principles of Serious Incident Management.
Source: Serious Incident Framework

The principles in Figure 19 are quite useful to us as a guide, given that NHS England has not produced a HealthCRASH Preparation Framework.

The plan should be Open and Transparent i.e. all those that either need or may want to see what's in it should have access to it. There's no point in this being buried in the deep recesses of the intranet where nobody can find it when they need it. It might be useful creating a Disaster Readiness section for HealthCRASH specifically and then making sure everybody knows where it is.

Ironically, when it comes to crises and indeed disasters in healthcare, we are not so good at openness and transparency. In early 2013, Mr Hunt was forced to introduce legislation in the wake of Mid Staffordshire, perhaps our largest 'lack of openness' scandal, to make data manipulation or misrepresentation a criminal offence. It is thus somewhat ironic that the very same Mr Hunt now stands accused of deliberately misleading Parliament and the public over weekend death rates and how they will be prevented by 7-day working, ignoring a specific warning over doing just that in the report itself.

In an SUI, there is the very important principle of taking action that is Preventative. Whereas that framework is predominantly focusing on ensuring the same thing doesn't happen again, our ahead -of-time framework needs to consider the most severe things that could happen and how to prevent them from happening at all.

For instance, I have discussed the impact of not being able to run the payroll and suggested how to prevent this scenario from occurring. I put it in Disaster Aversion because so much work needs to be done ahead of time. It isn't, however, the only disaster scenario that needs a preventative attitude.

Clearly patient care, including its quality and safety, are paramount. That much we will all know and accept. The Organisational Readiness Plan will need to explicitly detail what needs to happen to preserve this. To do just that almost certainly means identifying what we won't be doing that allows maximum focus on that.

This is an important concept that introduces two more principles; those of Proportionate and Timely & Responsive. A critical failing in many crises, allowing a disaster to unfold, is holding on to 'everything' for too long, consequently putting critical things at undue risk.

In the Ebola crisis, holding on to preserving local health service sensibilities meant that the real issues got dealt with much later than was advisable. I am not saying that those sensibilities weren't important, I am saying that there comes a point where other 'disaster preventing' stuff becomes more important.

This might look like a series of 'what if' scenarios that allow you to develop meaningful contingency plans for different circumstances. There isn't the scope here to explain what these might be but they will contain what you might immediately stop doing in favour of preserving something else.

Given my assertion that part of the issue we face arises out of our futile attempts to preserve everything we are told we should be doing, at the expense of sensibly addressing those things of greatest importance, I want to make one thing very clear. In case you were wondering, that does not mean being prepared to let go of financial performance in favour of clinical safety, although an adult consideration of just how willing you are to risk clinical safety for financial performance is absolutely a what-if scenario that needs considering.

It is clear that financial performance is a critical success factor for organisational and service security. What it is important to realise is that there are many other critical success factors too and a failure to recognise these and their chronological dependency is part of what produces the effect of lurching from one crisis to another.

It is worth remembering my *Upgrading our Thinking and Understanding* scenario that looked at complexity. It was a classic and highly repeated case of failing to understand what other critical success factors supported financial performance. A financial 'crisis' produced cost cutting measures (reducing capacity) that impacted flow, especially in elective care, which undermined financial performance - the strategy was self-defeating.

It is crucial that this Readiness Plan is constructed with a clear view of what needs to be preserved and how things fit together. Do you even know? Have you even thought about it? Do you have an explicit model to help prevent the scenario that I have just outlined? It is beyond the scope of this book to outline this in detail but you might want to access our framework for service security and stability, illustrated by Figure 20, as a good start.

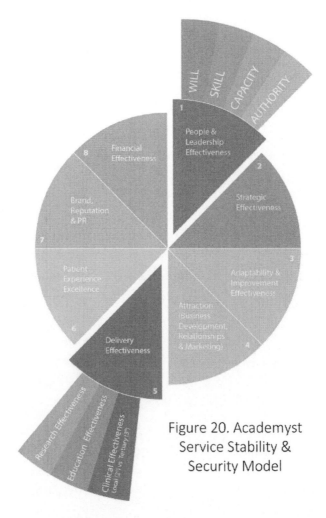

Figure 20. Academyst
Service Stability &
Security Model

You can download this framework without charge at:
http://academyst.co.uk/secure-service-model

The model outlines a series of critical dimensions and their relationship both to each other and the success of a service overall. Although it is focused on keeping services on the straight and narrow generally, it becomes an essential guide when times become tough. With Trusts, it is ignoring these chronological dependencies that has effectively produced HealthCRASH.

In case the strength or importance of this is not immediately apparent, I am saying that you have created your own nightmare, and collectively HealthCRASH, either by not having such a model or conceptual framework and/ or by not adhering to its underlying laws of nature.

By prioritising finance over some of the other stability-critical dimensions, you are doing the life equivalent of prioritising air over water, when nature is pretty explicit that BOTH are equally important to life. This simplistic approach to deeply complex problems is at the heart of HealthCRASH.

I realise that I have not conveyed the detail or specifics of what a good Organisational Readiness Plan, specifically for HealthCRASH, might look like. That was never within the scope of this book. However, I hope that I have conveyed the importance of having one and provided some principles that you may want to use when constructing you own.

Disaster Recovery - a Future View

If all has gone as well as could be hoped for, given the unexpected nature of challenge within a crisis or disaster, we may now be thinking that we might just get to survive long enough to clear up the garden after the maelstrom. Ironically, preparation for this starts well before we even enter the maelstrom and that is why I am covering it now.

My advice to organisations is straight forward, yet anything but simplistic. It is also positive, for you at least. Assuming you have averted as much as you can and prepared well, you have every possibility of owning the future i.e. a heightened level of success going forward. Why? Because sadly, the field will be clearer due to the demise of the less well prepared.

The People Component of Recovery

I want to reiterate something at this point that is fundamental to your future success. It is going to make uncomfortable reading because you have been behaving at complete odds with your own best post-crisis interests for quite some time now. It is in the realm of people and it is a consistent finding when examining factors impacting post-challenge organisational performance.

Consistent with our own Service Stability & Security Model (Figure 20), the organisations that do by far the best are those that are people focused and best places to work. This is illustrated clearly by Figure 21, for the US market.

Comparative Cumulative Stock Market Returns

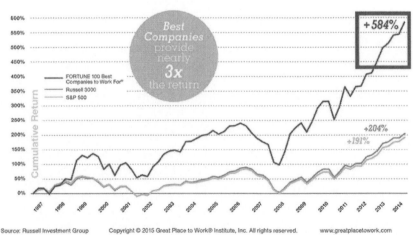

In case you were about to suggest that it is different here, this has been replicated in the Times 100 Best Companies to Work For in the UK and a myriad of other studies looking at the attributes of high performance companies or organisations, including the public sector. I am going to suggest ignoring it at your peril.

You can clearly see that in 2008, compared alongside other strong companies, best places to work and everybody else were all significantly impacted by the financial crisis. However, what is striking is the rate of return achieved post-crisis by best places to work. What's more, you could argue that the crisis was good for them because it is clear they are owning more of the future than before. They haven't just returned to their old growth track, they have gained a new, steeper growth trajectory.

I believe that the reasons are two-fold. First, the reason that they are still there is because their relationship with their staff saw them through. Strategies do not save organisations. People do. And I don't think I am wrong in saying you have been steadily killing yours in the interests of more-for-less, justified on the basis of the greater good. This was a poor understanding of your future and it has grave consequences.

The second reason is that when people are prepared to save an organisation they love (which they do out of their sense of ownership of that organisation and for leaders they respect - another wake up call, I am afraid), they will dig very deep for solutions. These organisations tap into the massive intellect and drive at their disposal. It is not predominantly the leaders that come up with plans, it is the people. The leaders support and direct them to innovate.

If you are thinking at this point "but I asked my people and they didn't do anything, and certainly not enough" then it is telling you just how much thinking upgrading you need AND just how much damage has been done to their relationship with their employer i.e. you. Uncomfortably, you might also want to reflect on what they might be thinking about you too.

Reiterating Service-led & Adaptability

Without going over already covered ground, I want to reiterate that my assertion that the service-led organisation is not optional is very much grounded in this understanding too. If you do not create the right working environment and culture, from top to bottom, you probably won't live to regret it, certainly not in HealthCRASH. That this transition is urgent, is much akin to the Captain of a submarine saying "perhaps we should close that forward hatch now" just as it is beginning to dive.

Your future will be very much dependent on preserving what you might need to rely on (people, need I say again, but not only people), whilst building much better, longer term solutions.

Adaptability will probably remain the most important critical success factor in part because we just don't know what will happen in our NHS as a whole. Thus, the form you need to take and what you might need to rely on is dependent on the future form our health service may take and I am cautious about using the word 'national' when thinking about post-HealthCRASH, as that would be an assumption I don't think we can make.

Readiness for a New System

In the absence of concrete information, we have to keep our options open and not risk things that we might need. You may well think that is very difficult in the absence of any indication from Government or indeed any suggestion from Government that they might even be considering a change of system. Ironically, it's really scary if they haven't (as it suggests a level of blindness, denial or delusion that we just should not have from Government), even though it's pretty scary if they have but have chosen not to mention it.

I, and other really intelligent observers, have had this debate for some time. Is HealthCRASH intentional, to create the conditions in which a Government could discuss an alternate system, or accidental, in which case suggesting a level of ineptitude (born out of denial, delusion and blindness) that is beyond scary for us as a population. It could be both. It can't be neither.

My personal inclination is that it is predominantly the former. Recent Governments have taken a strong interest in US health systems and the appointment of Mr Stevens himself, is some evidence of how much weight they place on that experience. If that is filling you with horror, knowing that the US health system is the most expensive in the world, we need to remember that it is not the most expensive to Government, given that until Obamacare, the US Government only provided healthcare (and in limited form) to around 18% of its population.

Rather than debating, whether this focus is a good or bad thing, a classic behavioural trap for us, we would be better thinking about what it is telling us about Government thinking in relation to the problems we have. I believe it is suggesting that perhaps they think they cannot afford healthcare for a population and are thus considering options, such as:

- Providing for part of the population
- Providing limited scope (even though they have said otherwise)
- Shifting responsibility onto other groups (Accountable Care Organisations)

We already have evidence in our system of a move towards ALL of these. What's more, they are ALL highlighting the importance of 'some' critical success factors that we would be best to acknowledge and preserve.

In each case, it looks like at least some, if not many, patients will end up with distinct choices to make, including about the location and type of organisation they wish to be cared for by and indeed the level of quality or cover they are willing to pay for. We may end up with a co-payment system, whereby patients pay something towards their care. We may end up with a system of basic state packages and enhanced packages for healthcare.

All of these point to the importance of quality, safety, accessibility, experience and reputation as enduring critical success factors. In a new system, our financial stability will come from being 'supported' by the system or by patients, or a mixture of both. They will support us because they want to and believe we deserve it.

Choice is already enshrined in the NHS Constitution. If that Constitution is enduring through HealthCRASH (and if you in any way subscribe to my 'intention' viewpoint then you'd have to consider that Government knew where the system might be going when they enacted that fairly recent constitutional change), then choice is here to stay and the critical success factors I have indicated are thus super-important.

I think a likely change, which is already in existence, is the increased importance of the Accountable Care Organisation. It is to this that I wish to turn some attention.

Accountable Care Organisations

Along with 'grip', the phrase Accountable Care Organisation (ACO) is firmly on all lips. We have multiple versions of this already in existence in our system.

The attraction to Government is obvious and unquestionable in its predicament of too much demand and not enough money. You assign the full responsibility for something, including all the money that is available for it, to a single entity that is now 'accountable' for the scope of what has been devolved. It's not new, not even to us.

Clinical Commissioning Groups (CCGs) are really ACOs. They are responsible for the provision of healthcare services to meet the needs of their patients, including paying the bills, irrespective of where a patient may choose to have care. They get a fixed, per capita fee for this and they are supposed to provide for pretty much 'all' of a patient's needs, accepting that some things are commissioned centrally too.

It is frightening how few truly understand this relationship. Each patient has a price on their head - allocation of funding on a weighted (depending on area and certain circumstances) capitation basis. Each patient must be a member of just ONE GP practice. Each GP practice must be a member of just ONE CCG. The CCGs budget for healthcare is essentially the head price x patients within the CCG's practices. And it isn't enough.

Until recently, the amount of money allocated for a patient's primary care was held separately. GPs are unusual. They run what I describe as a 'Membership Scheme' business much like a gym, in which they receive a fixed price (again with some weighting) for a patient, irrespective of how many 'sessions' they decide to attend. Much like a gym, the very best patient to have is one that pays the membership fee but then doesn't turn up for the rest of the year. Unlike a gym, these patients magically renew annually!

This is changing under the Five Year Forward View. On 1st April 2015, 64 CCGs and a further 87 in collaboration with NHS England, took on commissioning of primary care as well as provision of secondary care. Whereas there's a clear benefit in supporting integration, I am struck by the bravery of taking on probably our fastest failing part of healthcare. Of course it might not be bravery that has caused them to take it on. We will come back to this.

For some time, the Government has shown interest in what is called the Lead or Prime Provider model too. An example of this would be the award of 'all' musculoskeletal services in Bedfordshire, along with a fixed amount of money for them, to Circle Health. That contract value was £120m. That's £120m whether it's enough or not and that's very much the point.

Circle is now an 'accountable' care organisation for all MSK services in Bedfordshire. It is up to Circle to come up with a delivery model that fits the needs of those patients within that £120m figure. The Government is secure. The onus is on Circle. They have terms. They can't not provide and they can't stack patients in a line if there turns out to be more than expected.

An even bigger form of ACO is based on devolution. Recently, around £6bn of healthcare funding decision-making was devolved to Greater Manchester, a metropolitan council. This is enormously significant both for what it tells us and what it means for the future.

Firstly, it is a form of ACO. The rather complicated Board, representing 26 councils and commissioners, now needs to re-design 'Manchester' so that as a health and social care system it works. That's not an insignificant task, given that Greater Manchester has undertaken multiple attempts at reconfiguration as a health region and all have run into terminal difficulties. There's little debate that in current form it is almost impossible to sustain Manchester's healthcare infrastructure.

I would also like to point out that Manchester as a council has seen staggering cuts under austerity and this puts an enormous strain on social care, a vital part of the healthcare equation too. With health and social care funding now under the guidance of a single Board, and social care previously less protected and falling over faster, there is at least the possibility that this provides the mechanism for a raid on secondary care. It didn't escape me either that a largely Conservative coalition was devolving this £6bn to a 100% labour council.

There's no question that intelligent local design would be beneficial for healthcare. However, I can't help but think that this is far more about an 'impossible' future than an innovative present. Whichever way we look at it, our current Government is trying to 'devolve' responsibility for making the impossible actually work. This is a road that, once travelled, is very difficult to reverse up.

I am absolutely sure it isn't much of a leap to see what's happening as political protection in a scenario that is likely to have a less than palatable outcome. What's more, if it turns out well, the present Government can lay claim to the success of their devolution policy and if it goes wrong, perhaps their own underlying belief, then there is a 100% Labour council to put up for blame.

Despite this perhaps being immensely strong evidence that the Government itself expects HealthCRASH, I am inclined to think we need to understand what it means for healthcare providers in the future. Whichever way I look at this, one way or another, you will be one of two things:

1. An ACO

2. A Provider beholden to an ACO

Depending on your starting size, strength and aspiration, I would suggest this is as much a 'choice' as it is a likelihood. However, it is also very clear it is a choice with implications either way.

If you are the latter, then the health design you will need to adhere to is the one that the ACO leads the design of. If you don't like it, they are likely to simply say that they will then just find someone who does or who will comply with it anyway. Either way, your future is likely to be owned by a different 'boss', as the Government seeks to place distance between itself and the patient in terms of individual aspects of accountability.

I would strongly encourage you to think about what would make you an exceptional 'service provider' for a new type of ACO, as well as how you can build the right reputation and rapport with those that might be in charge. If you want a stark illustration of not entirely thinking things through, Bedford Hospital refused to participate in the Circle Prime Provider contract, choosing instead to reply on their capacity being needed and their service being supported by patient choice. It's a VERY risky strategy, given that Circle is in charge of the initial consultation.

Turning our attention to the former, it might seem like a double-edged sword. On the one hand, you get to design the system. On the other, you are left responsible if it doesn't work. Would you want to be Greater Manchester, knowing the history and likelihood of success? And they have responsibility for virtually all of the care, not just a specialty like MSK.

There is another consideration though that leads me to believe it might be a necessary evil of a choice. It concerns the crisis, if not disaster, that is already unfolding in primary care. As I see it, as primary care collapses in places, the burden of care will switch to secondary care organisations anyway, who can't cope already.

Consequently, I am inclined to think that a larger, hospital Trust may well be advised to become an ACO but with responsibility for primary care too. You might ask "why?" given the crisis in that sector. My reasoning is that you are going to end up with the fall out regardless, probably through already stretched emergency pathways and yet as long as you are a standalone provider your only option is to stand there and take it.

If you take on the ACO responsibility for primary and secondary care, it provides you with the opportunity to establish a complete re-design of the primary-secondary care structure. This may be necessary to come up with a new modus operandi that better manages the crisis in both. Lastly, as an ACO with primary and secondary care, especially if it includes community services too, you can re-design completely within your organisational boundary, rather than giving up funding and control to someone else. In effect, you can become your own System Architect.

None of these choices is easy and I have spent some time 'reflecting' on them as a way of encouraging you to think about what they mean for you, what is likely to be important, what critical success factors may be essential going forward and what choices you might want to make or prepare yourself for. These possibilities are far from the only ones and there are a myriad of unresolved anomalies.

For instances, we have commercial organisations with existing contracts, which limits the flexibilities an ACO might have. In effect, in an area where there are existing contracts, an ACO would probably have to take those on and honour them. That's a risk to an ACO, especially if they aren't good contracts.

I have suggested that patients will continue to enjoy choice, given its recently enshrined nature in the NHS Constitution. That also represents risk. An ACO might have to honour a patient's choices even if they are at odds with the ACO's interests.

If I had one piece of advice that I am wholly confident about, it is that I would not make the ACO decision or otherwise without a thorough assessment of what you'd be taking on, including the state of play of the players. For instance, if I was considering a patch with a number of poorly performing hospitals, with evidence of all of the failings I have described, I'd have to ask myself about the chances of being successful. It's asking for a very, very good risk assessment at the very least.

Owned by the Innovators

In the face of such challenging circumstances, I would suggest that the future will be owned by those with the best models and solutions to deeply complex problems. In effect, this will be those that step away from historical approaches with an open mind and a deep understanding of what's important, as well as the constraints at play. It will belong to the innovators.

I am proposing that the future will belong to those organisations that create the headspace and processes to support innovation. If you come up with a meaningful answer to a deeply complex problem, the system will welcome you with open arms. The future is yours.

The good news is that our healthcare organisations are full of innovators and individuals brilliant at coping with complexity. What's more, those same people have been rigorously trained to remain high functioning in the face of uncertainty (the backbone of good clinical care) whilst also taking a balanced approach to risk. If you never operated on someone unless the outcome was completely certain, you'd never operate. If you chose not to treat in A&E because you hadn't got all of the information and answers you felt were important, we'd have a horribly high mortality rate.

Ironically, that's the exact situation we have developing in our provider sector. Used to being told exactly what to do and knowing you are secure however that turns out has undermined the propensity to innovate and act proactively. As a businessman, I absolutely know that I will never have complete certainty. If entrepreneurs needed that to act, we'd have no new companies! So how do we cope?

Firstly, we trust in the expertise at our disposal. That's something that NHS organisations have to become re-acquainted with as a way of working. Secondly, we dig VERY deep in our quest to understand what's going on and, more importantly, where it's going - the direction of travel. Pitching ourselves with that direction turns a wild guess into a best guess and in an uncertain world, that's often as good as it gets.

However, there's a poorly understood aspect of entrepreneurialism that is going to become crucial to healthcare providers. Whereas following good leaders and innovators, as a 'fast follower' is a good way of living off someone else's highly innovative coat tails, in truth the future belongs to those that set the conditions for everybody else. They don't adapt to market conditions, they create them. I suspect, this will be as important in healthcare as anywhere.

These are organisations that don't defend against new delivery models, they create them. They don't discount new technologies, they seek out how they might use them to leverage how they work. Despite not having used the phrase, I hope you have already picked up that I am talking about the disruptive innovators. I believe you will have a choice in the future - learn to disrupt or accept being disrupted.

Innovation just doesn't happen miraculously. Google remains one of the most innovative organisations on the planet and it is worth looking at the lengths they go to in ensuring that innovation is a way of life, not an occasional piece of good luck. They invest in it. They recognise where it lies and what it takes to bring it out. It's true to say that many a healthcare provider recently has supressed innovation tendencies, or at least made it seem so difficult to realise an innovation that engaging in the practice is futile. I believe that is a mistake and one that needs fixing swiftly.

In Summary of Recovery

From the outset, I am going to say that without question, we will need a strong, resilient and committed workforce and so stop messing that up! If that sounds like a broken record by now then reflect on how important it is. I KNOW how much I am repeating myself and it is for your own good.

I know that it is easy to justify why you are making changes that fundamentally disengage them or drop their morale but rest-assured, feeling justified doesn't alter that course of action being equivalent to nailing your own coffin shut from the inside. The best strategy in the world is worthless if you have nobody to implement it and you have gone bankrupt in the meantime.

What's more, with such a committed, intellectually capable group of people at your disposal, I just can't see why you wouldn't want to tap into that. It contains so many of your answers. If they aren't behaving as you'd hope, it is because you haven't created the right conditions, NOT because they are at fault.

We are likely to be part of a new funding model for healthcare. The challenge is that we don't know what that model may be. However, I would suggest that we know enough or have sufficiently few potential scenarios that we already know some of the things that might be important and on which we may have to rely.

Our reputation is one of those things, whether we may be asking to be trusted to take on the responsibility for healthcare for a population or simply be a good provider to a different accountable organisation. We let go of reputation at our peril. Instead, I would already be seeking to enhance reputation in the arenas I am most likely or most want to succeed in.

A loyal following is another critical success factor, very much aligned with reputation but also reliant on other aspects too. What will we be known for and what will people's experience of us have been through HealthCRASH? Will they want to see us prevail, or will they be angry at what we have allowed to happen and thus more intent on helping others own the future?

Clinical quality and safety are both paramount and sacrosanct, along with our reputation and patient experience. Let's stop putting those fundamentals of future success at risk for financial reasons when financial recovery before HealthCRASH is an unlikely scenario anyway.

Do you feel more secure literally wrecking the inside of your organisation in so many dimensions to please erratic regulators in one dimension? Those same regulators will increasingly struggle to support you anyway and many of the strategies taken are undermining both your short term and longer term future. Be better than that. Dig deeper.

I want to round off my section of guidance for organisations by revisiting a much made statement or two.

Firstly, we live in an era where there has never been more opportunity but at the same time never more threat. Whether you benefit from the former or suffer from the last is very much a choice. It's a choice grounded in the quality of your thinking and the depth of your understanding, in both the system and behaviour. But then that's a choice too.

Secondly, in my lifetime, we will struggle with the putting the affordability of our healthcare system back inside the funding we have access to. It is going to get much worse before it gets better. As long as that condition remains, there is no reason why any one of you should fail but it is completely impossible for all of you to prevail. Survival is not down to luck (even if it helps). It is down to the decisions and actions you take. Those decisions and actions are underpinned by how you think and your depth of understanding, of both the system and behaviour.

As you reflect on my guidance, especially that last bit, you can be forgiven for having a sense of déjà vu. That's for a reason. Every problem you have today is more to do with your decisions, actions and approaches than the circumstances you have been faced with. If I am suggesting those circumstances are not only not improving but getting worse through HealthCRASH, then if you want a different outcome, you had better start thinking and acting VERY differently. I am sure you know what they say about continuing to do the same thing but expecting a miraculously different result.

Something magical will not just happen. Stop hoping for it and start recognising what you need to do. When you decide that's the road you'd like to travel, I'd be more than happy to provide a few pointers for the journey.

Individual Responses & Guidance

I am going to say from the outset that the implications of HealthCRASH and what an individual may be forced to do are much more difficult to discuss, in part because part of the solution for you may be part of the problem for your organisation. In protecting yourself, you may well exacerbate issues for your service and Trust.

Nothing is likely to seem morally or ethically a straightforward choice. Even within this chapter, I feel like I am personally, as author, without even being an employee, being asked to choose between organisation and individual. You will have ascertained already that I have been pretty hard on organisations as they try to solve their problems at the expense of, rather than through their people.

Perhaps to rationalise these issues more successfully, we need to consider this. A good organisation is one that seeks to behave in a manner that aligns the interests and well-being of the organisation, its constituents (you) and its patients, as well as perhaps system and commissioners too. We should be supporting good organisations.

The flipside of this is organisations who take courses of actions that seek to preserve the organisation at the expense of their people and even of their patients too, by undermining quality, safety and experience. They don't have to do this but they are choosing to do this. If they are choosing, then perhaps you should too.

Of course, life is never that clear cut. What happens if they are choosing but only because they don't understand or know what to do that's better? Shouldn't they enjoy your support?

This is a more difficult issue because I am still inclined to suggest that they should know better than undermining their own workforce. Perhaps it should come down to their willingness to seek out better options and to listen when things are going wrong. Both Mid Staffordshire and Barts Health opted for not listening and instead perpetuated a bullying culture and strategies at odds with their workforce's and patients' best interests.

One of those two organisations didn't survive to regret it and the other is currently recruiting a whole new leadership team to have another go. The recruitment adverts are asking for collaborative, clinically-engaging, far more transformational leaders who will drive change with and through their teams. I am under no illusions that they will have to work hard and fast to regain the trust of those teams after such a period of destruction but let's say that the jury remains out, at least.

Reflecting on Personal Consequences

I guess I am asking something very important that you personally need to reflect on; just how far are you willing to put your own health, happiness, marriage, career, professional integrity and well-being at risk for an organisation that doesn't seem to adopt the same commitment to you? Without a distinct decision in that, it is easy to end up sucked in to a point where the impacts are personally difficult to recover from.

Health & Well-being Consequences

If I asked you whether you would be prepared to give up your own health for your job, especially when you felt your organisation wasn't doing the right things, almost everybody would say no. And yet, in that HCSA survey that I mentioned earlier, 71% of those surveyed said that the level of stress they were under was taking its toll on their health. They reported effects such as:

- Exhaustion
- Depression

- Anxiety

- Gastritis

- Ulcers

- Raised blood pressure

These are real effects that they were already suffering and yet they were only 'thinking' about making changes. They were also reflecting marital issues, home issues and more. Very few were happy.

To be harsh (to be kind), maybe they were thinking if they did nothing, something magical would just happen. I know they were showing the sort of dedication and commitment that makes our medical profession the envy of the World but I am also concerned that they were also doing the one thing they say they wouldn't do when you ask them that very specific question.

Each individual needs to consider where they might draw their line. What are you prepared to risk out of commitment and how far are you prepared to go before deciding enough is enough?

There's no question that the choices will be deeply difficult to make. The timing will never seem quite right. It will always feel like a leap of faith into an unknown, even if the known is deeply uncomfortable (and proven to be so - a certainty). We all wonder whether it is 'just' about to get better and if we leap, will it be just too early and we'll regret it. I cannot change those feelings.

However, to balance those feelings, I am asking you to more accurately and deeply understand what's going on, seek out the evidence and objectively assess where it is going for you. I am going to ask you a very tough question, in the interests of balance.

You are going to constantly ask yourself a 'what if' question. When you get to the point of feeling like you've had enough, you'll ask "what if I make the wrong choice or do the wrong thing?" My balancing question is this; "what if you don't make a change when you genuinely should - where does that go, what's the price of that and how does it compare?"

Professional Consequences

It's easy to fall into the trap of thinking you are doing what you are doing out of professional obligation. It's absolutely true that we all have professional obligations and clinical professionals have a stronger more explicit code than most.

The GMC lays out very specific responsibilities towards patients, profession and the system in which you operate. You are required to protect all three. However, it is also worth reflecting on just how the GMC approaches the protection of all three through you personally. It's also the focus of revalidation and the backbone of Good Medical Practice.

Those two sacrosanct principles are keeping YOU in a condition that keeps the patients, system and profession safe, as well as acting with integrity at all times, for instance in speaking up when you have concerns.

Let me ask you what kind of shape are you in? Do you have enough time to do a professional and safe job? Are you able to keep up with a sensible level of professional development? Do you get sufficient mental and physical rest?

Being stressed, overwhelmed and exhausted, is highly likely to be the cause of errors, a causal link long established in the literature. If you look after yourself appropriately, you are less likely to have to worry about errors and the GMC. But what about integrity?

There are a myriad of reasons why errors and incidents occur and just as many of them are organisational, not individual. However, that doesn't mean they don't have individual implications. If the Mid Staffordshire disaster resulted in anything, it was the uncomfortable realisation that NOT raising concerns was not an option.

In ever stronger terms, we are told about the professional obligation to speak up. This is perhaps becoming even more important, given that the CQC has just been asked to model scenarios of a budget reduction of between 25 and 40% for the 2016/17 financial year. David Behan, the current CQC Chief Executive, is already warning of implications for its inspection regime.

Whereas some may breathe a sigh of relief at less inspection, I would suggest that it means we cannot rely on the CQC quite as much to pick up problems in a system that is going to have more of them. Quite apart from the apparent lunacy of weakening the failsafe mechanism at the most difficult time, it reinforces just how important professional integrity and speaking up are going to be.

This raises a further personal difficulty. Just because you speak up, it doesn't mean your organisation will listen or that you won't be personally vulnerable for apparently raising some inconvenient truths, perhaps inconsistent with the organisation's CIP plans.

In all of this, it is easy to draw the conclusion that you appear to be damned either way. However, I would suggest that the continued presence of the wrong behaviours by organisations is what presents the greatest personal risk. It creates that risk through your health and well-being directly, through errors and GMC issues as a more indirect consequence of exhaustion and being spread too thin and in creating impossible ethical and personal dilemmas internally.

We need to appreciate that we are hard-wired to mitigate personal risk. I am saying that as long as the organisation is behaving inappropriately, you are vulnerable - one way by challenging and another by not challenging. I'd love to call it differently but I think it comes down to a choice - and some vitally important strategies that you can adopt to reduce the personal impacts.

In any event, I'd recommend that all individuals need to learn how to raise concerns in a personally safe manner, whilst learning much better how to exert upwards and outwards influencing. It's not that these capabilities haven't always been important but they take on a personal safety importance in an era of erratic and dysfunctional behaviours.

You may also want to start drawing some lines now, around work-life balance, breaks, down time, professional practice and more. If I had one piece of advice right now, it would be to know precisely where your lines are in advance and commit to not stepping over them. It's the equivalent of going to an auction with a maximum price you'll pay and never a penny more. That keeps you safe. It's easy to pay dear when you have no explicit lines.

With this in mind, we need to turn ourselves to positive guidance - what should you do? As I unfold it across Aversion, Preparation and Recovery, you'll see the very difficult issues I have raised being tackled in hopefully a supportive and intelligent manner, accepting what I already said about nothing seeming quite perfect. If there was an obvious perfect course of action, you'd have already taken it.

Disaster Aversion

As we start into Disaster Aversion, it is worth remembering that we are discussing the aversion of a personal disaster - the steps we can take to ensure we don't suffer catastrophically from a health, well-being, marital and fitness to practice perspective. It is difficult to ignore though that a healthy organisation is an obvious answer to that.

Consequently, I will start with you and the success of the organisation in alignment. However, if you find yourself in an organisation that resolutely refuses to listen or adopt better approaches, we have to consider that aversion for you may run contrary to stability with the organisation. That's where the difficult choices need to come in.

Challenge Poor Choices & Strategies

I am going to start with your own depth of understanding, with some advice that is both vital and personal safety enhancing. Your organisation will be trying to make changes to improve its position or stability. Quite aside from whether they are taking the right leadership approach (which I have strongly challenged on earlier), they have obviously got to make sensible choices on what they are going to do. You will be asked to engage in their choices.

But how do you know they have made good choices? This will only come from your own depth of understanding and your ability to overcome you own internal mental processing. What have you disengaged from or opposed that was sensible? What have you supported that wasn't? How would you even know?

For all my criticism of the decisions and actions of Trusts at this current time, failing to understand complexity and what is in their future best interests, I am no less critical of individuals that perpetuate decline by disengaging from initiatives they don't understand but intuitively don't like. You may be right, you may be wrong but you are no more or less objective than the Trust you are resisting if you don't have a deeper understanding.

Consequently, this is my number one piece of advice for personal disaster aversion - understand deeply what is going on, why and how, so that you can genuinely recognise what's sensible, what isn't and how it might play out. This will allow you to challenge positively and contribute to an adult debate.

Your depth of understanding, along with learning to recognise and control the impact of your feelings and gut reactions, is paramount to leading with personal impact and influence. Your

Trust and system needs this to ensure that poor choices with adverse consequences are successfully exposed for what they are, so that better choices and more innovative solutions can take their place.

If you are confident of your position and understanding I am going to suggest that keeping quiet is not only no longer an option but paramount to allowing the conditions that precipitate a personal disaster to continue. However, we are surrounded by people saying they don't like one thing or another and we have to be personally better than that.

I recall suggesting the very same to the National Health Action Party, ahead of the last election. I asked what I thought was a sensible inquisitive question, along the lines of; I know that you oppose current Government policy, but what is your alternative suggestion to ensuring that we have a sustainable healthcare system, given its marauding unsustainability.

I have to say that I wasn't challenging their position or supporting any of the other parties. I was simply asking for clarity on what we would be pursuing, if we were going to abandon the current course of action. I didn't get an answer. I did get about a thousand Twitter notifications that left me wishing I'd never asked!

What I am suggesting here is that alongside challenging poor decisions, actions and indeed policies, we need to also be engaging in providing solutions, options and alternatives. Again, these will only come from having a deep understanding of the issue complexity but it is also a point of attitude.

It is easy to criticise someone else's poor choices, although challenge we must. But doing nothing is a poor choice too and to avoid this, we owe it to ourselves and our system to positively engage in designing better choices. Be better than just a naysayer.

Ironically, I am going to start the promotion of good thinking and leadership by suggesting you take a more active role in exposing the opposite. Part of the reason we have so many problems is that we have allowed poor thinking and leadership to go unchallenged. We quietly resist its impacts but we need to become better at exposing it for what it is.

The leadership approach adopted by many Trusts today is grounded on thinking that originated from the industrial revolution. It's not that this was poor thinking... at the time. However, the times were very different, the people wholly different too (in terms of intellectual capability and implicit power), and the nature of the problems being faced (mostly simple efficiency problems or poor organisation) had no relationship to the bigger picture, deeply complex problems that abound today.

Essentially, as these factors evolved, good organisations continually evolved their leadership approach, the NHS largely hasn't. Unfortunately, the leadership approach adopted was always unsuited to the healthcare environment. That's not just an opinion, it's an evidence-based observation, firmly illustrated by where we have managed to get ourselves to.

What's more, rather than learning from our errors, we seek to attach blame and then simply push even harder, still with the wrong approach. We lead incorrectly, we don't understand behaviour nearly well enough and we have completely the wrong structure and culture within many, if not most of our organisations. This leaves us inert and vulnerable.

We can all contribute to changing this most serious of conditions or traps. It involves exposing what we are being subject to much more openly, including the impacts that it is having. This latter point is crucial.

Many of your organisations almost certainly don't know any better. You may well question why we employ people who don't understand the leadership and transformation fundamentals, especially when we pay them huge salaries, but that doesn't alter the fact that we do. What I am saying is that changing this is a necessity as part of disaster aversion.

I am going to assume that you are still reading for a reason. I am going to assume that the rationale for HealthCRASH made sense, causing you to be concerned that we were bowling headlong into a disaster, whilst already being in a crisis. I am going to further assume that the advice for organisations made sense, causing you to want to read the guidance for individuals too, and so here you still are.

However, at this point, you could be at this very point for more than one reason. It could simply be that the advice made sense and so you wanted to discover more. However, I am more inclined to surmise that you thought the advice made sense but you see so little of it in active operation that you felt you needed the personal bit before it all goes pear-shaped. Am I on the right lines?

So, I am going to ask you a deeply uncomfortable question (for some, if not many of you). What have you done to promote the right things happening? What have you done to expose the wrong things that are currently happening? OK, 2 questions again but both are relevant.

If you read a whole bunch of things that you were worried about or that mirrored what you were seeing unravel in your own organisation, who did you tell about them? Who did you direct to read the same? Did you send it to Board Members suggesting you were worried that we were falling into many of the traps illustrated?

Equally, if the advice made sense, did you send that around more widely too, suggesting that there were answers and suggestions that could help?

I know, I am being slightly unkind because you are still reading. Who advises 'everybody' to read a book before they get to the end? However, I am being very serious about exposing both the poor thinking and leadership we have whilst promoting better approaches. Consequently, I believe you now know what to do (if it makes sense)!

I actually believe, for all my assertion of the inevitability of HealthCRASH, we are at a crossroads, where the turn we take is the tipping point. At the time of writing, we are just ahead of the 2015 Autumn Spending Review. Everyone is wondering what is going to happen. I think we already know and I suspect it is the wrong turn.

If the CQC have been told to model cuts of between 25 and 40%, Health Education England are battling over the protection of their training budgets, we are reducing public health budgets, 80% of acute Trusts are in the red and worsening but being told to get a grip' and almost 'everything' is being 'safely' devolved onto someone else's plate, I don't think we need the Spending Review to see where this is heading.

But, what if, suddenly, everybody could see what was going on for what it was? What if the house of cards was suddenly visible? What if the true state of our organisations was visible at this deeply important time? What if the lack of transformation capacity or capability was unignorable? What if the true gap between funding and stability was exposed to everyone, by everyone? I don't think it risks anything because on current evidence there isn't really much to risk - where we are headed is why you are still reading. However, it might just cause enough people to stop and think that it helps avert a crisis turning into a disaster.

So, what are you going to do about that?

If we are going to lead ourselves to safety, we have got to understand that it starts with holding our organisations and the system to account. That's an active thing. You are not doing so by reading and agreeing but not openly sharing or supporting. One person saying something struggles to change anything but one of one million people, saying the same things is unignorable.

If one aggrieved doctor can start a petition that attracts 223,000 signatures and causes a debate in parliament on a vote of no confidence in Mr Hunt, then each of us has a very important role to play in disaster aversion for our organisations and system and in so doing, averting disaster for ourselves also.

Contribute Positively to Good Organisations

That leads me into my next suggestion - positively engage, step up and play your part.

I am not going to regurgitate the very large section on organisational disaster aversion through more appropriate leadership, structure and transformation that I have outlined earlier. However, I do want to spend some time on your role within that.

I want to say straight out that this isn't a suggestion for everybody to step up in all circumstances. Quite the opposite. I am going to suggest it is a conditional offer.

If, as you share or contribute to better thinking or solutions and expose poor thinking or plans, your organisation seems to be wanting to learn and dig deeper, THEN it is time to step up. What I am saying is that if your organisation shows the necessary humility and contriteness to understand the error of its recent ways, then it has the potential to seize the future with confidence and take you with it. It can't do that without you.

This is quite a turning or tipping point for you as an individual too. Why? I am sure you can see the sense in going the extra mile for an organisation that wants to be a survivor for the right reasons but what happens if it doesn't show that tendency?

You'll notice that in their reactions to your holding them to account. You'll see the evidence in their behaviour. Do they say 'thank you' for bringing this to our attention?

As an optimist, I am hopeful that it produces a sea-change in behaviour in the right direction. As a realist, I suspect that this type of response will come from the few, not the many. If you hear about the "the circumstances" or "we tried all of that" or "everybody else is doing what we're doing" then you have a very important piece of behavioural evidence that suggests that disaster aversion probably needs to be individually focused, not organisationally.

So, what does 'positive contribution' really mean? At a simple level, it means dropping the 'them and us' language or position and realising in a good organisation it's just 'us' and we need to work collaboratively together with a shared sense of purpose.

Mahatma Gandhi said, provocatively but not less pertinently for today despite its historical nature; "we need to be the change we wish to see in the world" and that means being 'big' enough to start that process yourself knowing that not everybody will follow suit immediately. The point is, it has to start somewhere.

From an organisational perspective, this behavioural tendency is captured beautifully by the guidance in *Managing Oneself* from the late and brilliant Peter Drucker in his seminal article first published in 1999 and available still in Harvard Business Review.

He said that we can no longer rely on our organisation's decisions and actions alone to create stability and success for us and that means "*we have to learn to develop ourselves. We have to place ourselves where we can make the greatest contribution to our organizations and communities. And we have to stay mentally alert and engaged during a 50-year working life, which means knowing how and when to change the work we do.*"

What can you lead? What can you participate in? What can you improve? What ideas do you have? What do you need to learn? How can you ensure you understand, deeply? How can you positively contribute to others understanding?

Ironically, I don't think I am suggesting anything that doesn't already happen in clinical medicine. Everything on my little list is part and parcel of being a successful doctor or nurse. We don't share ideas, new discoveries and write only if we are being paid explicitly to do so, do we? We don't only improve stuff because someone gives us a bonus or a merit award, do we?

We do make sure we are always keeping up to date though. We do approach our work with humility, in case we are wrong. We challenge our own decisions, action and perceptions. We hold each other to account because we know it is important. We do volunteer for responsibilities and we do respect good leaders who are nurturing and inclusive.

All I am saying is that if we want this to turn out differently i.e. avert disaster, then it will be as much in the contribution we make as in the profound realisation by organisations. However, we do also need to be 'allowed' to make a difference and hence my earlier decision-point.

IF the organisation seems to want to do the right thing, then support it and step up. If it doesn't, then it is time to look at some personal disaster aversion and preparation and accept that the organisation isn't going to provide it. As you will see only too clearly, there's a fine line between disaster aversion versus preparation and it is mostly about your propensity to act proactively and when.

Health & Wellbeing Disaster Aversion

To consider what appropriate disaster aversion or preparation might be at an individual level, we might want to spend just a few minutes thinking about what we are trying to avert or prepare for, individually. What could happen to us as an individual? The most likely disaster impacts will fall into one of the following three areas:

- Health and well-being loss, including home problems and divorce

- Reputational and professional damage, including GMC Fitness to Practice issues

- Financial and career loss, frequently the same thing without appropriate preparation

Let's start with the first two, given that both are mediated through the position your organisation puts you in, or which you allow to emerge. I have spent enough time on asking you to reflect on what these might mean to you and how prepared you are to allow that to happen.

I have made it very clear that the very first aversion strategy is having a distinct position or line in the sand beyond which you will not go for your own personal and professional well-being.

It is important that you draw that line in the right place and be confident in drawing it, so that you know when to legitimately say no. I see too many individuals saying no to things they shouldn't whilst allowing other organisational atrocities to slip by without notice.

Part of the reason that this is so important is that once you arrive at that line and say 'no' you will find that your organisation's attitude to you will change too. Nobody wants to be there and that's why we agree to a level of pressure that we know is unreasonable. However, as we have discussed, there comes a point whereby the consequences of not addressing the pressure are greater than the consequences emerging from your organisation's changed attitude. You need to make sure you are ready for that and that means being assured that your line is in the right place.

Employers have obligations under the The Health and Safety at Work etc Act 1974 and the Management of Health and Safety at Work Regulations 1999 to ensure the health safety and welfare at work of their employees. This includes minimising the risk of stress-related illness or injury to employees. It doesn't matter whether they are a healthcare organisation or otherwise. Employment law stands.

However, whereas falls hazard or unmaintained and faulty equipment is easy to assess, an employer's culpability in not looking after your mental and functional health is less straightforward, not helped by everybody's stress tolerance being different anyway. However, that doesn't absolve employers of their responsibilities, or you.

This is a huge topic area and well beyond the scope of this book. It is also a fast-moving topic in which I am not an expert, although I am fully aware of my obligations as a director.

Your organisation is obliged to do two key things that are paramount. One is to provide a working environment that is safe and the second is to address good faith safety concerns without victimising the person raising them. Safe includes mentally safe, not just physically.

They are supposed to conduct a proper and formal risk assessment and especially at times of change. My experience is that this is not the norm, or not the norm when considering stress, even if the organisation says it does. However, employees have a duty to take reasonable care over their own health and safety and of others who may be affected by their actions.

Consequently, employees should:

- Inform their employer if they feel the pressure of the job is putting them or anyone else at risk of ill health

- Suggest ways in which the work might be organised to alleviate the stress

- Inform their employer if they are suffering from a medical condition that appears to be long-term and is affecting their ability to carry out day to day tasks, including memory and learning (stress counts!)

- Discuss any reasonable adjustments that could be made to assist them in performing their job (including more support, more breaks or less work)

My pragmatic advice is to do two things to ensure that you are drawing your line in the right place:

1. Seek medical advice and get real over what 'stress' really is and if you are medically diagnosable already with stress

2. Engage with the relevant and helpful bodies on what would constitute an unsafe or unreasonable load i.e. likely to lead to safety or stress-related issues

If you don't want to go to your GP, you can always start with Occupational Health. However, if push comes to shove, you need the back up of someone in 'higher authority' than your line manager or organisation. You cannot be discriminated against for health reasons. It doesn't mean you won't be, it just means you have some comeback if you are.

There are a myriad of official bodies and helpful organisations that will offer advice if you are genuinely concerned. Some of them end up picking up the pieces of problems that occur. My suggestions, in no particular order, include:

- Health & Safety Executive
- British Medical Association
- Other Unions e.g. Unison, TUC etc
- Occupational Health
- Medical Defence Union
- Medical Protection Society
- Royal Colleges
- Employment Solicitors (good ones)

All of this allows you to draw a line, confidently in the right place. However, there's an additional consideration and I have seen organisations use it. It is possible that at some stage they may suggest that it is not their environment that is at fault but your ability to cope with it i.e. you, not they, are at fault. It's one of the reasons we find it so threatening - we know this can happen.

My advice is to ensure you plan intelligently, prioritise sensibly and know at all times what you can, can't and aren't doing and why. It won't stop them from trying this approach but you do need to have something to fall back on to demonstrate you are doing things in the right way, competently and it is the workload at play, not your time management.

The goal of disaster aversion is to avert a disaster. That sounds obvious to the point of being pointless in saying but just how many individuals wait until they have a disaster e.g. a heart attack, before taking action. You do not have to wait that long and you should not wait that long.

By arming yourself with what's reasonable and what isn't, supported by one or more third parties with influence, you can draw a safe safety line and refuse, politely but firmly, to step over it. I know that will feel difficult and unpleasant. But will it feel as unpleasant as a heart attack, or losing your licence?

Before finding yourself at the line, you need to raise your concerns with your employer. They are obliged to take them seriously. It doesn't mean they will. However, you need to be in the position of raising your concerns as to the potential for harm asking them to conduct a risk appraisal (another obligation) and do something if they find something. That doesn't mean they will.

As you come closer to your line, you need to be raising these concerns with more frequency and more strength. They need no chance to wiggle through by saying "we didn't know" and you need to make sure you document these occurrences, not just say them.

As you approach your line, you need to be prepared to do two things.

One is to not step over that line but to tell your employer about the action you are taking not to e.g. to close beds to reduce load.

The second is to invoke the support of one of those other third parties to support you. For instance, if you are genuinely worried about safety, both yours and consequently the patient's, then asking the MDU or MPS for support is a good place to start (given they pick up the negligence claims), as well as Health & Safety Executive, who uphold adherence to the rules and laws.

I am going to re-assert that arriving at this point will be one of the most difficult and unpleasant experiences you will face professionally. I can't make it any less so. However, you are doing this to avert a personal disaster and that is important to keep in mind.

Trusts constantly rely on the vocational nature of healthcare and your unwillingness to challenge because of how threatening it feels. Ironically, this tendency in you has perpetuated their tendency to keep pushing on with more-for-less to the extremes they have. I am not going to criticise you because I know how tough it is to face this. However, I am going to say that there comes a point when enough really is enough, or you might have an even bigger disaster on your hands.

Employment & Career Disaster Aversion

Of course, the very best way to remove your source of work environment risk is to remove yourself from that work environment i.e. leave. I started with an approach to manage to the load because my inclination is that underneath all of this you like your job and probably have a pretty embedded life wherever you are based.

After we have worked for many years in one place, moving feels like a very scary thing to do. Additionally, we have spouses and children to consider. The latter may be doing A-levels and the former may have their own career to think of too.

So, with that in mind I am NOT suggesting that you move, only that you consider moving if the alternative is a personal disaster from a health and well-being perspective i.e. to avert disaster. There is an additional circumstance too.

I have spent a great deal of time reinforcing just how important it is to more deeply understand what's going on and how your organisation is behaving in response. You need to know not only what state your organisation is in but which direction it is travelling and why, as well as whether it is showing any tendencies towards humility and learning i.e. adopting a better approach. All of this is for a very important reason and it is about timing.

If your organisation is showing distinct signs of failing and very few of improving, then you need to consider what that failure would mean for you as an individual. This is very much tempered by your length of service and age.

For instance, if you are two years off retirement, with 35 years' service under your belt, in a non-Foundation Trust, it is quite possible that the right strategy might be protecting your health and well-being whilst waiting for the organisation to fail and take redundancy, or compensation. That is not going to be quite as attractive if you are 32 and have 2 years' service with this organisation.

I am again going to say that I am not an employment specialist and advice is the right way to go. Ask the question; "if my employer went into administration tomorrow and ended up closing, laying me off in the process, or cutting my service to save itself, what would I be entitled to?" You can then weigh that up against other options.

I want to stress again that disaster aversion is about taking action before a disaster. If you can reliably predict a disaster, fairly early, you have the ability to prepare and create other options. That time is invaluable, depending on what you want to do. For instance, if you wanted to work abroad, there are visas to apply for, certificates to get hold of and more. If you know this ahead of time, there is little lag between something happening and you being ready. Let's consider some examples or suggestions, all of which I have seen undertaken.

The simplest is a move to another employer. Hopefully, armed with what I have provided so far in this book, you have everything you need to assess whether you are jumping out of the frying pan into the fire. The only thing worse than losing your job unexpectedly is losing your job unexpectedly when you are brand new i.e. with no protection!

Increasingly, I am seeing individuals reduce that risk by moving out of this healthcare system. Scotland has a system much closer to our pre-existing one but it is true to say that it also isn't so stable and the weather is undoubtedly colder. There are other places to move to.

Australia and New Zealand have very well-regarded healthcare systems and lots of older UK synergies, making the personal transition easier. Depending on where you go, the weather is likely to be better and the quality of life a quantum improvement, accepting that depends on what quality of life you have here. Canada is another work-life balance positive choice, although its healthcare system too is pressured. Where you go in Canada is an important choice.

There has been an enormous growth in Middle Eastern healthcare systems and they are determined to grow western-modelled approaches. They are frequently very well-funded and more inclined to trust the professionals they employ to set up and lead strong departments. It's why they are so keen to have western professionals. However, there are obvious life-style considerations too, depending on where you go, some of which are not compensated for by higher, tax free salaries.

These are not the only off shore possibilities. I have seen people go to the Caribbean, which is often a step back in health system 'organisation' but comes with much better weather and the excitement of being part of something that is developing. I think much depends on what you are interested in and it will come down to a risk-benefit analysis and that's why you need the time. You don't want to be emigrating to Dubai on a whim. It needs planning and it needs careful assessment.

Another choice is to set up or help set up a new provider aligned with the healthcare system's direction of travel. It has never been easier to do so but it comes of course with risk and obligations. Again, you need time to assess this and very much consider if this is you.

Depending on the nature of what you do, you can seek out someone else who wants to do this. You can lean towards healthcare provision and let them be the entrepreneurial drive. You can see, however, just how important it is to have that deep level of system understanding, to ensure you make good choices and do something that has legs and longevity.

Modern thinking GP practices or groups are certainly seeking to bring secondary care services into primary care settings and tend to do so as separate businesses. They need secondary care professionals to do the work and are frequently interested in joint ventures.

If you are in a vulnerable secondary care service and your Trust isn't listening, you could consider seeing if some of the local GPs are interested in forming a new business. Again, you can provide the expertise and they can, very successfully in many cases, provide the business acumen, fund raising capability and operational drive to make it successful. They also have existing premises, which can limit risk enormously!

Aside from emigrating or setting up on your own, my last primary piece of disaster aversion is in ensuring that if disaster strikes, you have options. Whereas a little financial stock-piling wouldn't go amiss, I am primarily referring to your reputation and capability. It is for this reason that I stated so early how dangerous it is to allow that to be undermined. It's your fall-back.

If you believe that the next few months or years could see your job at threat due to service or organisational failure, you need to be planning and preparing now for that eventuality. Having a plan and knowing what you'll do is half of the battle.

What do you want to be known for and how will you develop that reputation? What else do you need to study, clinically, leadership, business or otherwise to give yourself options and make yourself attractive, if not invaluable, in a choppy climate? Taking Peter Drucker's advice, what are you interested in that you could become an expert in for someone who needs it?

Part of this work is starting to build your presence and your network. Do people know you? How externally active are you? Who are the people you need to know and be connected to? It's an unfortunate irony that the very conditions that might warrant you to be building an external reputation also happen to be conditions that tie you inside your organisation more and more.

I haven't even begun to scratch the surface on options, which is reassuring too, of course. I might suggest that almost everybody starts to develop 'something' that they can fall back on. It doesn't have to be salary or career replacing but it can be disaster re-assuring, knowing you have something meaningful to do that you could ramp up.

We are building some clinical educational initiatives that could well provide a platform for some. The UK is renowned for our medical education and depth of clinical expertise. It's a good example whereby someone (us) provides the entrepreneurial drive and you provide the clinical expertise.

It's also an example of practising what I am preaching. If the NHS enters HealthCRASH, my own leadership and transformation training interests may be adversely affected, regardless of this perhaps being the very time they're most needed. I am not naïve. I may hope for the best but I am inclined to plan for the worst as well.

My wife is a senior doctor in a historically stable and successful Trust, running a department that tends to be cash positive for the Trust. She is deeply committed to her employer but she is not complacent either. She has a coaching practice around interviews and careers and she has training interests too. She would be heart-broken if something happened to her job because she loves it. She's also mindful of the need for a plan B. In troubled times, it's potentially good advice for everybody.

Disaster Preparation

As you have probably gathered, much disaster aversion also seems to look very similar to disaster preparation. I am not going to argue the point. It's a semantic line between the two.

However, I have previously made the point that it mostly comes down to the propensity to act, early. If you can determine the likelihood of a collapse in your organisation at the hands of HealthCRASH, then disaster <u>aversion</u> would be seeking gainful employment or alternative occupation elsewhere, possibly 10,000 miles away.

If the issue of collapse and disaster, or personal loss if it happens, is less clear cut or you'd like to see how it pans out anyway, then disaster preparation is perhaps a better option. Even still, there's a tremendous overlap and sometimes the only difference is whether you have pressed the 'go' button.

With that in mind, this is a much shorter section because I do not want to revisit all of the same ground. However, instead, I do want to concentrate on how you might prepare to be 'in' a disaster, rather than avoid one.

First off, I am going to do some reiteration. However, it will have a new flavour too.

I want you to imagine that you come into work one morning and without any warning you are called to the Executive Suite. They sit you down and offer you tea. Consequently, you know it isn't good news.

Unknown to you, until this moment, discussions have been going on behind the scenes to reduce costs in a 'Trust survival' way i.e. by closing something major. Your service has been running at a loss and is strategically not the top choice for preservation in a Trust that is quite shoot-from-the-hip anyway. They are going to serve notice to the commissioners on its closure. Just like that.

Let me ask you a question. What is it that's in place for you that you could simply shake their hands, thank them for your employment up to now and calmly walk out leaving them wondering what just happened? That's what we mean by preparation.

It wouldn't be that the news was good. You wouldn't be working here if it wasn't at least attractive to do so. I would suggest that it was a plan B, something that meant that this was not a shock or disaster but simply the occurrence of a potentially possible event that effectively pressed the button on your plan B.

What plan B is we have covered at some length already in the section on personal disaster aversion. The only difference between the myriad of options suggested there and here is that you didn't press the button. If your decision was to wait and see, you still need to engage in the options investigation and appraisal process, just not with the same propensity to leap.

Disaster preparation is not about leaping. It's about waiting until you need to leap and knowing exactly what leaping looks like so that you can step right to it, not least because you might not be the only individual leaping and thus, being ahead of the queue might be important too.

It is quite appropriate to have a number of options on hand and indeed even a short term option and a longer term one. They all need to be eyes open options.

Financial Preparation

Depending on your circumstances, you might need to prepare financially. Whereas having a plan B is clearly in part a financial preparation exercise, it isn't the only consideration.

The degree to which you need to financially prepare, actively, will depend on the answer to the following question: If I was made redundant tomorrow (my service closed, notice was served etc), what would this mean to me financially, when I consider my personal circumstances, liabilities and obligations?

Of course, that answer depends on how severe and how long you think the effects may last and that is also dependent on the presence or absence of a good plan B, including how long it takes to implement it. If you are expecting to take 6 months to find another job in a specialty with little prospect for locum or bank work, then 6 months is what you have to plan for or consider.

Let's say for the sake of argument that this scenario would produce some financial discomfort, where it is a threat to normal existence or simply an erosion of a valued lifestyle. Preparation is knowing how you would cope, including what steps you might need to take ahead of time.

At the very least, it's a heightened awareness of what gets spent where and when, including what the implications of not spending it are, or possible alternatives. You may think I am off territory (or even the reservation here) but I am raising it because at the point of disaster, you are highly likely to lose some of your cognitive control and so the work you do ahead of time is crucial to sensible action within a disaster.

An example might be that a month into say 3 months' notice, your mobile company calls up and offers you a replacement handset for simply agreeing to stay with them. You had no intention of moving anyway. However, agreeing to a financial commitment of say £50 per month for 2 more years limits your option of just letting go at some point. What if you might consider going abroad? You don't want a £1,000 bill at a difficult time just because of a weak or, more accurately, unprepared moment.

I am sure you might be inclined to say "sure, I'd have thought of that" and you may well be right. However, I am also saying that it is easy to say that now, when you are not faced with that notice but then all sorts of limbic, cognition-fuddling processes start to kick in. It's one of the reasons I say to organisations that they need to prepare ahead of being in a disaster.

The construction of a decent spreadsheet with all spend listed, quantified, risk assessed and alternative identified, along with nett earnings and your plan B options is very much financial preparation 101. You can start using it to take financial preparation decisions right now. Examples might include:

- Paying off credit card balances in preparation
- Negotiating an overdraft facility, just in case
- Switching investments from long tie-ins to more instant access e.g. an ISA
- Seizing good moments to liquidate shares
- Holding fire on things with sizable, longer term commitments or heavy liabilities

The list is not exhaustive and I don't want anybody going off selling shares on this advice. I am saying that as you head into this very turbulent period, know what's what and take your financial decisions with this in mind too.

To be able to do this effectively, you also need to know what the financial implications are of one decision versus another. For instance, it would be easy to 'jump' employment early without discovering that you would be better to be made redundant. Over my earlier years in industry, I have seen that play out quite commonly.

If you are going to be 'let go' or believe you have reach a point of no return, you can often negotiate a settlement instead of a lengthy legal process. If that's what's called a COT3 agreement, negotiated through ACAS, or compromise/ severance agreement, then part of it can be tax free. That can make a big difference. You'd be advised to know what's possible and what's not in advance.

This is a highly technical area and so it is worth seeking professional advice. In case you are thinking that's an unnecessary expense, let's remember, you are only here because of your assessment of the likelihood of this becoming a reality. In which case, it's hardly unnecessary and could save you thousands.

Emotional Preparation

I have alluded to an issue that will be an important one. If you genuinely believe that HealthCRASH is a probability and that your organisation may suffer, some of which may rub off on you, then you need to be very mindful that this will adversely affect your thinking and decision-making.

Everybody believes that it won't. Every day, we judge how somebody acted under stress and espouse how we would have acted differently. The difference is that you are doing this from a position of calm rationality and even detachment and they were in the thick of it.

Much like my aforementioned advice on mastery of thinking and feelings being akin to learning how not to react when a patient hearing bad news throws a wobbly, preparing ourselves for being the person receiving bad news takes much the same form. The key is in preventing limbic processing from overwhelming our ability to put a pause between stimulus and response.

By far the most effective strategy for this is to build up a series of what-if scenarios, including what they would mean, how you could expect to feel and what you would need to do that is sensible. That mental preparation is worth its weight in gold. It forces thinking over just feeling-driven behaviour. It forces you to exercise active judgement, not passive reaction.

We do know this, of course, we just aren't used to exercise this in HealthCRASH and its consequences. The principles are the same but we forget the principles because the context is different.

I bet most of you would never send an angry email directly in response to receiving one that made you angry. You might write it but then delay sending it until the next day and it usually then needs a big re-write! That's good - a step between stimulus and response. However, I also know that every one of you HAS done it at some point and some of you fall into the trap frequently. Yes, it's all right, we all know. You can admit it.

The point is, even with a little strategy, it proves difficult to do sometimes. The better we get at exercising the cognitive 'restraint' muscle, the less likely we are to take courses of action that we later regret.

Almost everybody is going to be subject to scenarios and decision-points that require intelligent judgement but at times or in circumstances that are perfect at creating quite the opposite. What if your Trust puts a load of jobs at risk as part of a re-grading exercise? I have seen people leave when their jobs were secure, I have seen people stay, knowing they will get re-graded and knowing that they can't afford to live on the new figure. Both are examples of limbic behaviour.

Given that we are considering preparing for a personal disaster, such as a job loss, there is another form of preparation that is just as important and my latter example leads into it nicely. If you are going to be 'let go' then it is important that you do that also!

The point at which you know that your future does not reside with this organisation is the point at which you need to switch over to Disaster Recovery i.e. building your future. You will retain certain obligations but that's a long way from what you will have been doing as a deeply committed employee. You need to minimise your commitment down to the essential bare minimum and use the time to engage in building.

What initiatives can you hand over early? How do you prioritise your patient care from your other work? If you are doing over the normal hours (bet you are...), how can you bring that back inside the work time you are being paid for? It's too easy to find yourself working even harder in this period out of commitment to an organisation that has just demonstrated and indeed cemented no ongoing commitment to you!

This happens because you'll have a stressful conversation about being let go and everybody will then want to feel better. This is a vulnerable time for you. You may well set the tone and agree to things that produce this very effect. In doing so, the meeting ends all smiles but that brief moment of weakness has cost you valuable re-building time.

Better would be to negotiate what you can get out of, given that they are letting you go. A good example is to ask whether you can have some time off or an earlier finish in exchange for 'working really hard' to get your job in order now. That provides a legitimate mandate to rapidly get things squared away, leaving you more time to work on you!

Disaster Recovery

It cannot have escaped your notice that much disaster recovery has its seeds sown in aversion and preparation. However, there are new points to be made and things to reiterate.

Having taken the approach to separate individual and organisational interests in this personal section, based on you helping organisations that try to do the right thing and being prepared to protect yourself or even walk away from the others, it is worth briefly re-visiting recovery as a re-intertwined activity.

If the organisation has adequately averted and prepared, then you will currently be helping it build a more stable and successful future. If that's the case, it will almost certainly be a service-led organisation and the relationship you have with it will be very different to the strained relationship of late.

You'll be amongst a resolute group of individuals, with a devolved, trust-based structure and culture, with strong internal collaboration and a commitment to innovation and a new approach. You'll be mitigating further effects, improving things and exploring opportunities to seize. I sincerely hope that this is where you find yourself.

There is every possibility that it has not turned out that well and in which case we need to consider what you might be doing and what you might need to start today that puts you in the right place for swift disaster recovery at a personal level.

Preserving Recovery Faculties

I hope I have made the point about personal health and well-being strongly enough that this isn't what we need to discuss from a recovery perspective. If you are near-dead, with no confidence left and a track record of high sickness and absence, you aren't in great shape for recovery.

Equally, if you became so emotionally-driven, distant, withdrawn, angry and indeed absent, you could well have risked your marriage and personal relationships. You will not be so driven to recover if you do not have the same things to drive for. All I am saying is that you need to protect these aspects of life above all else.

Why do I keep reiterating it? Because protecting the above requires some of our hardest choices and most unpleasant experiences in the moment. Consequently, us mentally frail human beings are more inclined to justify that it won't happen to us just because we don't want to face the more immediate challenge of tackling it, with all that brings.

So, I make no apologies for the constant reminders, even if I acknowledge that's it's tough to keep being reminded. I'd rather you acknowledged this most severe of risks and were a little annoyed at the reminders than deluded yourself into thinking "not me, someone else" and then paying the ultimate price. Look at the HCSA survey, if you need a reality check.

That said, I know I have been strong in these assertions and that you are still reading at this point suggests you are taking the warnings seriously enough. Consequently, I am more inclined to think that recovery is likely to be about finance and career.

Key to this is the reputation and capability you hold, along with the tendency to be a first mover, or certainly not a laggard. Much of my aversion and preparation focus was about being ready to press a 'go' button and a compelling and productive alternative.

Nature says that you don't need to be the fastest to survive, just a reasonable amount faster than the slowest. However, it's also true to say that the faster ones do get the choicest meat, as well as those that operate as a group. With that in mind, todays actions could be classed firmly as further preparation but I see them as disaster recovery because by their very nature they suggest you are doing something different and that has probably been stimulated by something not going so well.

To be perfectly clear about this, rapid recovery is underpinned by the following:

- A compelling alternative
- That you can do successfully
- That you can start doing at the very moment that disaster becomes a reality i.e. the first point of real need

Clearly so much depends on what you have chosen as a plan B (along with potentially a plan C, plan D etc). However, apart from the practical things like a visa to work abroad, along with a Certificate of Current Professional Status etc, I want to reinforce the faculties that are enduring no matter what.

Your compelling alterative comes from your reflection, your deepening understanding, your monitoring and your careful construction of a plan B. I have paid this out already. However, to do all of that requires time. The challenge is that sometimes we just don't have that time until we have lots of time on our hands i.e. after a disaster!

Time is a hugely valuable commodity and we need to preserve it. It's a core reason for better, more in control time management because not only does it help us maintain our boundaries from a well-being perspective, it allows us to discover how best to create that plan B and discover what it ought to be. You cannot afford to not have the time to produce your compelling alternative. Headspace goes alongside that time. Prioritise both.

As you start to go through that process, you may well discover that there are new skills you need. Apart from these also requiring time to develop, this must go into your recovery plan.

As an example, if you intend to build work as an independent healthcare provider through Any Qualified Provider, you are going to need to know how to get a licence to practice when it isn't covered by your employer. At the same time, you may well need some business and marketing skills too, or you will be allowed to provide but have no work!

Reputation is crucial and the last example reinforces that. It's just as important when working for someone else. You need to preserve it with all your might - you don't want a fitness to practice case on your CV. Equally, when you know what it needs to support, you can start assessing whether it stacks up.

You need to be able to adequately answer the question; why should these patients want to come to me, or why should this GP practice want to recommend me, or why should this employer in Australia want to employ me specifically? If you can't think of a reason, then they won't either.

Even if you can think of the reasons, I would encourage you to ask yourself how they might know that. That is asking you to think about the visible evidence of who you are and why you are great at what you want to be doing. If that evidence isn't there - BUILD IT!

Recovery Networks

Whatever our healthcare system looks like today, it will be different tomorrow, possibly radically different. Our system is evolving all the time but HealthCRASH has the potential to change it radically, with new principles and potentially brand new delivery models and relationships.

Besides thinking through for yourself, by building your understanding and interpretative abilities, developing networks with other new thinking, fast moving individuals is crucial. Not only will you move further, faster by learning to build ideas and evaluate possibilities together, you may well need help in building whatever you choose to build.

I made a fairly strong case that the future will be owned by the innovators. What happens if you just aren't that creative? Will you be left out? You don't need to be. Innovators need more detail-focused and operational delivery people in much the same way that these latter groups need the creativity of the innovators. Networks are an important part of your future in a system that is redrawing the lines.

Who are the like-minded individuals you'd feel proud to work with in building a new, stronger, more resilient health system the other side of HealthCRASH? Why would they want you? What knowledge, skills, insight and capability do you bring to the table? How will you develop your reputation to ensure that they find you and when they do, they want to join with you?

I talk about innovators as though these are individuals. They could just as likely be companies or existing providers or other healthcare organisations. I have suggested that some will find this a time of immense opportunity and others a time of tremendous threat. That you are engaging in this section suggests you may at least be worried your organisation is in the latter category and not looking likely as a future leader.

However, that doesn't mean that the Trusts today will all disappear. We can't 'replace' a secondary and tertiary care infrastructure with all new players although we could replace each and every one of those with new leaders and indeed new 'owners'. New leaders building a new system will undoubtedly need good people who can support the design and implementation of that new system.

I guess I am saying that perhaps we need to be less focused on the bricks and mortar definition of a healthcare provider or Trust and more mindful of who may be running these organisations, along with how. The buildings may be the same, the way they work and how care is paid for could be completely different. It could be a model that has much more integration. It could have more independent providers. We would be ill-advised to see these options as mutually exclusive.

The growth of the Accountable Care Organisation is a case in point. The ACO is potentially a new leader. The leaders in ACO-healthcare models are primarily US-based. However, even there, there are a multitude of different ACO models, stretching from highly integrated delivery systems such as Kaiser Permanente to the near-opposite VPOs - Virtual Physician Organisations - smaller, independent practices that come together to engage in larger scale activity or contracting.

As if to reinforce this reality, only this month (October 2015), we have seen 35 West Midlands GP practices, involving 150 partners, come together into a 'virtual' healthcare partnership, headed by a highly forward thinking, former Acute Trust CEO. That's a group with a great deal of potential power, whether existing organisations like it or not. I'd be watching closely.

Whether you'll be wanting to rebuild a career with a forward-thinking innovator or possibly be an innovator in the new system, it's clear that knowing the right people and having the right networks will be crucial.

I would round off by saying way too many people have spent the last few years seeking out like-minded people who will support their largely misguided case for staying the same and abandoning policy. Regardless of the disasters lurking in some of those policies, I am inclined to think that the smart money has been on thinking about the future, not hanging on to the past. And the really smart money has been working out who those future thinkers are and joining with them in one form or another.

As you can see, none of these questions or pieces of advice are answered by something you can 'just do' tomorrow if you found yourself on the wrong end of a disaster. Consequently, it seems entirely appropriate to start building today. Hope for the best, plan for the worst is a good mantra. I'd like to update it to; Hope for the best, plan for the worst but plan for a successful future out of whatever unfolds, disaster or otherwise.

My final advice in this arena is about you and why they, the innovators and innovating organisations, would want to engage with you. You may not have the skills they need at this point in time. However, I am inclined always to remember what a good friend reminds me of constantly. He says "recruit for attitude and train for skill".

This is important advice if you are on the other end too. People will want you for your thinking, your attitude and your understanding, along with your propensity to engage in a positive future. With so many naysayers around, you could just stand out rather prominently by upgrading your thinking and contributing to that future in many ways beyond your clinical capability.

It's all there for the taking but you have to want to, be prepared to and understand how. As with everything then, Disaster Recovery is more a decision and frame of mind than it ever is about luck or longevity.

In Overall Summary

I have presented a rationale for HealthCRASH. It was never about what I think or persuading you of something. You have to decide and you need to make sure for yourself.

My singularly most important piece of advice is that if you think there is literally 'any' possibility that I am indeed correct (and I have given you some pretty clear evidence and many ways to consider it), then your next action should be to confirm for yourself the data and evidence necessary for you to be sure about your own conclusions.

Why? Because the next step must be taking meaningful action to ensure you are secure. You shouldn't contemplate doing that by trusting me because I don't have to live with the consequences of what you choose to do. You do. You also have to live with the consequences of choosing not to act too.

Whatever you do choose, you will want to be making choices from a position of confidence or certainty and that requires evidence and understanding. Regardless of HealthCRASH or otherwise, your future success is underpinned by that.

Some of you will believe I am right and yet still do nothing, unfathomable though that is. I would love to be able to change that but I accept that it will always be a reality. I truly hope that circumstances treat you kindly and that luck is on your side, even though I wouldn't recommend it as a strategy.

I would also like to reassure you that it is never too late to do something meaningful. The passage of time may increase the severity of the circumstances whilst removing some of the easier or more beneficial options but it doesn't render you without any. If you find yourself in that position, I will hopefully be able to and certainly gladly offer guidance at that point.

My stronger encouragement though is that regardless of 'hope for the best' being your default strategy, learn to plan for the worst even if you don't press the button. These times are different and I think we all know that. They require a different approach to normal.

For the rest, who want to act or feel that they need to, regardless of whether they want to, I hope I have offered some guidance and indeed some hope. We live in a time where there has never been more opportunity but never more threat too. Success, or failure, is a choice, not a chance, even if some chance comes into it. If you decide you want a better future, I'd be delighted to try and help. Don't be a stranger.

For organisational leaders I would urge one thing above all else. Take a long look in the mirror and ask yourself a vitally important question from a position of internal openness. That question is; *do you feel genuinely confident in what you are doing and how it will turn out, or is that just a convenient form of denial because to consider otherwise is personally so very challenging, deflating and downright scary?*

If you answer yes, I wish you the very best and I genuinely hope that you are right. However, if you are brave enough to conclude that you aren't so sure - that perhaps you haven't got enough answers, even if you have some - I would offer this encouragement; that conclusion is actually a turning point in the right direction taken by the strongest of leaders.

You have just opened yourself to discovery, without the baggage of having to maintain an outward face that is frankly worthless if it all goes pear-shaped. If you are prepared to turn that corner, then I will offer my promise and commitment to helping you discover what needs to be done. I am not remotely naïve or egotistical enough to believe I have all of the answers but I am quietly confident I have many of the right questions.

To round off a synthesis that started life as an article but ended as a book, I am going to turn to some wise words by an enduring and successful leader, Jack Welch, former Chief Executive of GE. Most importantly, he said "When the rate of change on the outside exceeds the rate of change on the inside, then the end is near"

We are entering a period of considerable and accelerating change at a time when our organisations are most dead in the water. If we are to invest in just one thing that improves everything, it will be our capability for rapid, intelligent transformation and adaptability, based on massively upgraded thinking and understanding.

Our future rests not on the magnitude of challenge but in how we respond. That is our shared purpose - to respond intelligently but rapidly. I think the next step is down to you. What are you going to do, next?

(a page of guidance and suggestions follows this one)

What Next Guidance

You may want some reminders and ideas about what to do next. So many simply file it under 'interesting' but I'd like to think you are going to DO something meaningful.

TELL EVERYBODY

If this book and its conclusions resonate with you, then shouldn't 'everybody else' know about it to?

Who do you value & respect who would appreciate the heads up?

Who needs to read it because they have a position of influence?

Who really needs to read it because they are part of the problem (don't tell them this)?

- Send them all the Amazon link
- Share it on social media
- Just tell them about it

PROVIDE A REVIEW ON AMAZON

I'd be delighted to hear your feedback and it would help other potential readers too. Simply go back to the product page and leave a short review and rating, warts and all.

TELL ME YOUR THOUGHTS

I mentioned it in the book but I'd love to hear what your reflections were. Here's a little reminder of where to go to leave them:

http://healthcrash.co.uk/my-view-on-healthcrash-likelihood/

ASSURE YOURSELF

My strongest recommendation is be secure about acting. You need to assure yourself, not just trust me. That's a big detective process but there's a helpful short cut below too.

DEEPEN YOUR UNDERSTANDING

My key piece of advice – understand and evolving system and learn to exercise much better judgement. We can help in this:

http://academyst.co.uk/insights

FOLLOW THE HEALTHCRASH STORY

Keeping up-to-date is a real challenge. We started a website especially for this and you can sign up to receive updates. We'll try our best to keep up for you!

http://healthcrash.co.uk/

About the Author

Mr Andrew Vincent MBA DipM
Partner, Academyst LLP
Head of Leadership & Transformation

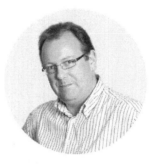

I am genuinely passionate about really making healthcare work. Increasingly it isn't but absolutely it must. I have spent the last 15 years passionately devoted to that purpose.

I bring to the table a long and deep understanding of our emerging healthcare system, including the complexity of issues it faces, how this is likely to change over time and what it means for individuals, services and Trusts. However, it is my behavioural expertise that most pertinent, when understanding why we have the issues we have and why we don't seem to be able to get out of them.

My provocative and challenging stance comes from the firm belief that we approach leadership almost entirely at odds with the evidence base and behaviour, yet everything we need to know to literally transform the stability of our system is known but not applied. We can and must do better.

I have an MBA with Distinction from Manchester Business School and I am an Oxford University Press author, besides a self-published one too. I have 15 years' experience specifically working with individuals, services & Trusts in improving leadership, adaptability and collaboration effectiveness, following a more operational career all the way up to director level, budgetary responsibility to £100m+ and international experience of many other healthcare systems.

I would prefer to be judged by substance, not CV, however experienced & knowledgeable I may be.

Printed in Great Britain
by Amazon